SPORTS OPHTHALMOLOGY

SPORTS OPHTHALMOLOGY

Edited by

LOUIS D. PIZZARELLO, M.D., M.P.H.

*Assistant Clinical Professor
of Ophthalmology and Public Health
Columbia University
College of Physicians and Surgeons
New York, New York*

and

BARRETT G. HAIK, M.D.

*Professor of Ophthalmology
Tulane University School of Medicine
New Orleans, Louisiana*

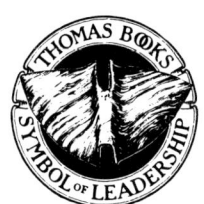

CHARLES C THOMAS • PUBLISHER
Springfield • Illinois • USA

Published and Distributed Throughout the World by
CHARLES C THOMAS • PUBLISHER
2600 South First Street
Springfield, Illinois 62794-9265

This book is protected by copyright. No part of
it may be reproduced in any manner without
written permission from the publisher.

© 1987 by CHARLES C THOMAS • PUBLISHER
ISBN 0-398-05309-X
Library of Congress Catalog Card Number: 86-29997

With THOMAS BOOKS *careful attention is given to all details of manufacturing
and design. It is the Publisher's desire to present books that are satisfactory as to their
physical qualities and artistic possibilities and appropriate for their particular use.*
THOMAS BOOKS *will be true to those laws of quality that assure a good name
and good will.*

Printed in the United States of America
Q-R-3

Library of Congress Cataloging in Publication Data
Sports ophthalmology.

Includes bibliographies and index.
1. Sports ophthalmology. I. Pizzarello, Louis D.
II. Haik, Barrett G. (Barrett George) [DNLM: 1. Athletic
Injuries--prevention & control. 2. Eye Injuries--prevention & control. 3. Sports Medicine. QT 260 S78576]
RE827.S66   1987   617.7'13   86-29997
ISBN 0-398-05309-X

CONTRIBUTORS

David H. Abramson, M.D.
Clinical Professor of Ophthalmology
The New York Hospital/Cornell University Medical Center
New York, New York

Marcel Amyot, M.D.
Associate Professor of Ophthalmology
University of Montreal
Montreal, Canada

John K. Davis
Adjunct Professor
Pennsylvania College of Optometry
Philadelphia, Pennsylvania

George S. Ellis, Jr., M.D.
Assistant Professor of Ophthalmology & Pediatrics
Louisiana State University Medical Center School of Medicine
New Orleans, Louisiana

Barrett G. Haik, M.D.
Professor of Ophthalmology
Tulane University Medical School
New Orleans, Louisiana

Eugene M. Helveston, M.D.
Professor of Ophthalmology
Indiana University School of Medicine
Indianapolis, Indiana

Frank Hoefle, M.D.

Associate Clinical Professor of Ophthalmology
Columbia University College of Physicians & Surgeons
New York, New York

Barry D. Jordan, M.D.

Clinical Fellow
The New York Hospital/Cornell University Medical Center
Department of Neurology
New York, New York

Pierre F. Labelle, M.D.

Associate Professor of Ophthalmology
University of Montreal
Montreal, Canada

Cynthia Mackay, M.D.

Clinical Instructor in Ophthalmology
Columbia University College of Physicians & Surgeons
New York, New York

Richard A. McDonough, IV

New York, New York

Sally Moore, M.D.

Associate Professor Clinical Ophthalmology
Columbia University College of Physicians & Surgeons
New York, New York

Hugh M. Moss, M.D.

Assistant Clinical Professor of Ophthalmology
Columbia University College of Physicians & Surgeons
New York, New York

Louis D. Pizzarello, M.D., M.P.H.

Assistant Clinical Professor of Ophthalmology & Public Health
Columbia University College of Physicians & Surgeons
New York, New York

Contributors

Calvin W. Roberts, M.D.

Assistant Professor of Ophthalmology
The New York Hospital/Cornell University Medical Center
New York, New York

Alain P. Rousseau, M.D.

Professor and Head
Department of Ophthalmology
Laval University
Quebec City, Canada

James A. Salisbury, M.D., P.A.

Morganton, North Carolina

Bernard J. Slatt, M.D.

Associate Professor of Ophthalmology
University of Toronto
Toronto, Canada

Harold A. Stein, M.D.

Professor & Chief of Ophthalmology
University of Toronto
Toronto, Canada

Raymond M. Stein, M.D.

Cornea Fellow/Wills Eye Hospital
Philadelphia, Pennsylvania

Wayne M. Whitmore, M.D.

Clinical Instructor of Ophthalmology
Cornell University Medical Center/The New York Hospital
Assistant Attending Ophthalmologist
Manhattan Eye, Ear & Throat Hospital
New York, New York

*We would like to dedicate this book to
our families*

PREFACE

GOOD VISION is an asset to any athlete. Regardless of the sport, performance is effected by the level of visual function and keyed to its maximization. The demands of each sport necessitate development of specific visual skills. Acuity, visual field, and stereoperception are just some of the elements of a well-developed visual ability. A good athlete uses all of these facilities to the utmost.

As each sport makes specific demands of an athlete's vision, so too are ocular injuries sport specific. Preventative measures, when tailored to a sport, can successfully save many eyes from injury.

This book addresses these two elements of vision in athletics. For each sport discussed, vision maximization measures such as spectacle and contact lens correction are described, as well as protective devices and measures that will not interfere with the performance of the sport. Early chapters will discuss basic eye anatomy and physiology, acuity, and stereoperception as well as basic treatment of ocular injuries. Subsequently, each of the major individual and team sports will be discussed in detail by expert ophthalmologists with extensive personal experience in their respective fields. This book will serve as a useful reference for physicians treating athletes of all types.

We are particularly indebted to Anne Kirsch for her editorial assistance. We would also like to thank Robert Woolley for artistic work. And none of this would have been possible without the secretarial assistance of Helen Moriority, Lorraine Gattuso, Patricia Lapinski, and Alice Krysiewicz or the support of the Benjamin Fund of Southampton Hospital.

CONTENTS

Page

Preface xi

Chapter

1. VISUAL PHYSIOLOGY — *Hugh M. Moss and Sally Moore* 3
2. LENSES FOR SPORTS VISION — *John K. Davis* 9
3. COLOR VISION — *Cynthia Mackay* 45
4. FOOTBALL — *Eugene M. Helveston* 51
5. PUGILISM — *Louis D. Pizzarello and Barry Jordan* 65
6. AQUATIC SPORTS — *David H. Abramson and Richard A. McDonough, IV* 71
7. VISUAL APPROACH TO WINNING TENNIS — *Harold Stein, Bernard Slatt, and Raymond Stein* 81
8. AVIATION OPHTHALMOLOGY — *Wayne Whitmore* 111
9. BASEBALL OPHTHALMOLOGY — *Frank B. Hoefle* 123
10. GOLF OPHTHALMOLOGY — *Calvin Roberts* 133
11. THE EYE AND SHOOTING — *James A. Salisbury* 139
12. WINTER SPORTS: HOCKEY AND SKIING — *Alain P. Rousseau, Marcel Amyot, and Pierre F. Labelle* 149
13. SPORTS EYE INJURIES: FIRST AID PREVENTION — *George S. Ellis, Jr.* 171

Author Index 187
Subject Index 191

SPORTS OPHTHALMOLOGY

CHAPTER 1

VISUAL PHYSIOLOGY

HUGH M. MOSS AND SALLY MOORE

WHEN MAN evolved from the early hominids and wandered into the savannahs after the Ice Ages, he moved on two legs and acquired several remarkable adaptations. One was physical endurance achieved in part through a large surface area of hairless skin containing sweat glands. This enabled him to become a superb hunter capable of running his prey to exhaustion. Another was the development of unprecedented eye-hand coordination.

In addition to the development of technologies and civilizations, man has indulged his superb eye-hand coordinations in sport. Many modern sports involve fast moving objects. Skilled play requires a high level of perceiving, judging, anticipating, and moving. These are among the most complex of sensori-psychomotor reactions.

The sensory arc of eye-hand coordinations is vision, but not simply vision as it is usually tested. The dynamics of play are far removed from the ophthalmologist's office. The routinely tested functions of visual acuity, refraction, accommodation, fusion, stereopsis, visual fields and color vision may indicate a fundamentally sound visual system. However, the detection of motion, generally untested, is of critical importance in sports involving high velocity missiles. The skilled athlete, using minimal visual clues and instantaneous judgment, anticipates the final critical position of the missile and his response to it.

Microelectrodes in retinal ganglion cells have revealed that retinal receptors are most sensitive to contrasts. Empirical awareness of this has led to the use of white baseballs, chartreuse tennis balls and black pucks. In football, no serious attempt has been made to standardize a high contrast ball, in part because concealment is at least as important as visibility.

Cerebral cortical cells have been shown to be sensitive to stationary linear stimuli at the "simple" level and to movement at the complex and hypercomplex levels. A remarkable revelation of this Nobel Prize research by Hubel and Wiesel was that the mammalian cerebral cortex appears to be highly sensitive to the contours and movement of a stimulus apart from its exact retinal position.[1] This sensitivity is not confined to the peripheral retina. The entire retinal surface is uniformly sensitive to movement.

Good central visual acuity may be important to the athlete under certain circumstances. Early and subtle visual clues such as the facial expression of a distant opponent are valuable. Hoefle has called attention to the relative importance of visual acuity to a baseball outfielder compared to a pitcher.[2] To avoid losing a hit ball, the outfielder must see the initial trajectory of an object subtending only five seconds of arc, while the pitcher need only count fingers at sixty feet. However, movement of an image on the retina at velocities of a few degrees per second degrade visual acuity. Whether or not a player wears refractive correction, either glasses or contact lenses, is an individual decision to be entered into by the athlete, the eye consultant, and the coach. Few athletes should be advised to consider surgical reduction of myopia by radial keratotomy because of possible healing delays with fluctuating vision, and because of the unknown risk of future eye trauma.

Sensory fusion and stereopsis are of doubtful importance in the skillful performance of the most popular American team sports. Experienced clinicians know that patients who have grown up with an amblyopic eye demonstrate no incapacitation in eye-hand coordination. This also applies to patients who have strabismus, with or without amblyopia. Strabismus present from a preschool age is generally not associated with diplopia because of suppression. The scotoma of amblyopia is most often monocular and central with peripheral vision intact. The scotoma is overlapped by the visual field of the sound eye.

Athletes have reached high levels of professional performance despite an amblyopic eye. Wesley Walker, a wide receiver for the New York Jets and an NFL All Star, catches passes over his shoulder on the same side as his poor eye, amblyopic from a congenital cataract.

The principle concern of the ophthalmologist in the early treatment of amblyopia is to provide the patient with a functional second eye. It is disastrous when a patient with an amblyopic eye develops a serious injury or disease of the only good eye. In only a minority of patients does the treatment of amblyopia result in normal binocularity. Some degree of suppression of the involved eye, to which the patient has adapted, usually persists.

Sudden loss of vision in one eye is considerably more incapacitating than a lifelong amblyopic eye. Adaption to monocular status can take months and full confidence may never be restored for the athlete. Dave Bing, a former all star guard for the Detroit Pistons, suffered a retinal detachment and subsequently returned to play, but apparently with less than his former confidence.

Protective eye wear is advisable in all sports where the eyes are at risk, but are of critical importance to the athlete with only one good eye. Kareem Abdul Jabar, the great center of the Los Angeles Lakers, wears protective eye wear because of recurrent corneal abrasions.

Sudden onset of diplopia is also incapacitating and virtually always sidelines an athlete. Occluding one eye eliminates the diplopia, but involves the slow adaptation from binocular to monocular vision, often over months. Because acute diplopia is usually incomitant, prisms are only rarely a satisfactory solution for an active athlete. Scott Eaton, a former wide receiver for the New York Giants, was sidelined in 1972 after closed head trauma resulted in a superior oblique paresis with intractable diplopia.

Young children adapt quickly to diplopia through a mechanism of almost instantaneous suppression. Adults lack this facility but over time, tend to become less aware of the second image. This adaptation appears to be a function of how intently the patient maintains awareness of the second image as against awareness of other objects in the visual field.

Retinal disparity between the two eyes, the basis of stereopsis, decreases with distance. Stereopsis is five times more sensitive at two meters than at one hundred meters.[3] Clinical tests for stereopsis such as Polaroid® and random dot stereograms reveal a latent period up to several seconds before stereopsis becomes optimal under stationary circumstances. For the quarterback spotting a receiver downfield or a basketball player shooting a jumper, stereopsis has a role secondary to more instantaneous visual cues, such as contrast, size, and shading.

The eyes move to scan the terrain, to fixate a moving object, to follow its flight, to converge on its approach, and to stabilize the image during head movement, all in coordination with other bodily activities. These functions all have definite limitations that can be taxed in sports involving high velocity missiles.

Saccadic eye movements are the most rapid and serve to change foveal fixation. Voluntary saccades are mediated from the frontal lobes. Involuntary saccades are the fast phase of jerk nystagmus. Saccades achieve velocities up to 700 degrees per second.[4] The sensory system cannot cope with such rapid movements, so that a form of visual suppression occurs during saccadic eye movements.[5] Thus, the eyes are not seeing during the brief moment they are refixating.

Compensation for this interruption of vision is provided by slow pursuit eye movements which serve to maintain the image of a moving target on the fovea. These are mediated from the occipital lobe. Pursuit movements are relatively slow, up to about one hundred degrees per second. While a tennis ball or baseball travels as fast as one hundred miles per hour, humans cannot track faster than fourteen miles per hour.[6] With practice, athletes learn the various trajectories of a ball. From pursuit during the initial phase of the trajectory, the final position of the ball is anticipated.[7] Bahill found that batters from the Pittsburgh Pirates were able to track a pitched ball over only the first 30 percent of its trajectory from the pitchers mound.[8] "Keep your eye on the ball" is advice that cannot be literally followed.

Vergence eye movements, that is, converging on an approaching object and diverging on a receding object, are the slowest of eye movements. The reaction time for fusional vergence movements is about 160 m/sec, and for accommodative vergence movements, about 200 m/sec.[9] The vergence itself takes as long as one second to complete. Hubel has shown that batters do not use vergence eye movements which are not needed to track a ball from sixty to six feet.[10] The pitched ball is too fast.

Vestibulo-ocular reflexes maintain clear vision during head rotation. Through stimulation of the semicircular canals, eye movement is produced equal and opposite to head movement. The vestibulo-ocular reflex is more sensitive than smooth pursuit. This can be demonstrated by the observation that a printed page is more blurred when it is moved quickly side to side, than if the page is held still and the head is moved.

The otolith mediates a modest counter-rolling of the eyes. This cyclotorsion is limited to the first six degrees of head tilt.[11] Disturbances of the vestibulo-ocular reflexes, such as nystagmus with oscillopsia, can be totally disabling to an athlete.

In summary, while a routine eye examination can detect the presence or absence of gross flaws in the visual system, it does not explore all of the complex and self-compensating mechanisms of the athlete's visual system. Stereopsis is not of critical importance in the most popular American sports. Athletes can do well with good vision in only one eye, however, it cannot be overemphasized that anyone with only one good eye must be protective of it.

REFERENCES

1. Hubel, D.H., and Wiesel, T.N.: Receptive fields binocular interaction and functional architecture in the cat's visual cortex. *J Physiol (Lond), 160:* 106, 1962.
2. Hoefle, Frank: Baseball ophthalmology. In Pizzarello, Louis D. and Haik, Barrett (Eds.): *Sports Ophthalmology.* Springfield, Thomas, 1987.
3. Ogle, K.N.: *Researches in Binocular Vision.* New York, Hafner, 1964, pp. 133-141.
4. Leigh, R. John, and Zee, David S.: *The Neurology of Eye Movements.* Philadelphia, Davis, 1983.
5. Campbell, F.W., and Wurtz, R.H.: Saccadic omission: Why we do not see a grey out during a saccadic eye movement. *Vision Res, 18:* 1297, 1978.
6. Schalen, L.: Quantification of tracking eye movements in normal subjects. *Acta Otolaryngol, 90:* 404, 1980.
7. Jones, Michael J., and Melville G.: Dependence of visual tracking capability upon stimulus predictability. *Vision Res, 6:* 707, 1966.
8. Bahill, A.T.: Keep your eye on the ball. *Welcome Trends in Ophthalmol, 5:* Aug. 1983.
9. Hubel, D.H., and Wiesel, T.N.: Receptive fields binocular interaction and functional architecture in the cat's visual cortex. *J Physiol (Lond), 160:* 125, 1962.
10. Bahill, A.T., and LaRitz, T.: Why can't batters keep their eyes on the ball? *Am Sci,* May-June: 249, 1984.
11. Adler, F.H.: *Physiology of the Eye.* 4th ed. St. Louis, Mosby, 1965, pp. 457.

CHAPTER 2

LENSES FOR SPORTS VISION

JOHN K. DAVIS

WHEN ANY PRODUCT has a sports connotation in its name or advertising it is endowed with an aura of quality, durability and superior performance. Family sedans are advertised as "sports sedans" or as having sports car characteristics. Running and hiking shoes are worn full time for their support and comfort. The Airforce Flying Sunglass has resulted in a generation of "aviator" sunglasses and prescription frames that rarely leave the ground.

Sports lenses, then, should be of the highest quality, and designed not only to perform well in their intended use but in other uses where they might be worn. Participation in a sports activity implies an effort to perform well. Whether it be driving, cycling, baseball, or racket sports, a high level of visual performance is required. The optical design and quality of lenses for these activities should be controlled to enhance performance if possible, and detrimental effects should be minimized.

Many sports activities involve exposure to glare, excess visible and ultraviolet radiation. The color and density of tinted lenses and their ultraviolet transmittance contribute to the visual performance, comfort, and safety of the wearer. There is scarcely a single activity, in sports or out, that does not expose the wearer to possible eye injury from mechanical impact of some kind. For some sports, particularly racket sports, a prime reason for wearing lenses is protection against mechanically imposed injury. Other sports may not uniquely require mechanical protection, but prescription lenses or absorptive lenses worn to enhance visual performance should be able to withstand anticipated impacts. They should not add to the risk of eye injury.

Protection against injury should have top priority. It should be the dominant requirement in lenses designed for sports use. Let us consider first the characteristics of lens material and design.

LENS MATERIALS AND THEIR IMPACT RESISTANCE

Prescription lenses, sunglasses, sports glasses, and industrial safety glasses are supplied mainly with one of three materials. These are glass (treated by heat or chemicals for impact resistance), allyl resin (commonly known as CR39,® a trademark of the P.P.G. Industries, Inc.), and polycarbonate.

Polycarbonate is a newcomer to the ophthalmic field but has long been used for military visors and industrial masks. Its impact resistance is spectacularly superior to that of the other materials. Its chief drawback is that it must be coated with an abrasion resistant coating. The coated polycarbonate, however, has an abrasion resistance superior to uncoated allyl resin and comparable to coated allyl resin lenses.

Dress prescription lenses are available in chemically treated and, rarely, heat treated glass, allyl resin and polycarbonate. There is no minimum thickness requirement, but they are usually supplied with at least a 2 mm center thickness. Glass sunglasses are often mass produced and heat treated. They may be slightly less than 2 mm thick. Sunglasses are also available in allyl resin and polycarbonate. Some are formed from molded or laminated plastic sheeting. There are tinted over the counter products labeled "sports glasses" or "shooting glasses," however, these products are often no more impact resistant than ordinary sunglasses. Fortunately, there are some sports sunglasses and shields available in polycarbonate that provide wrap around protection and adequate impact resistance. It is necessary to read the labels to determine the materials, the intended use, and the standards met by these glasses.

Industrial safety plano spectacles, goggles, and prescription lenses are available in heat treated glass, allyl resin, and polycarbonate. Some "sports" or athletic frames are available for these lenses. Special protectors for racket sports and other high-risk sports are becoming available. Again, the manufacturers' labels should be read carefully with respect to material, intended use, and adherence to standards.

The Industrial Safety Standard Z87.1 1979, and current revised drafts, require a minimum thickness of 3 mm for all materials. The exception is polycarbonate eye shields molded in an integral front, covering both eyes. These can be 2 mm thick (Appendix II).

Since glass, ordinary plastic (allyl resin), and polycarbonate are all used in the complete spectrum of eyewear which may be used for sports activities, the suitability of these materials should be evaluated for each individual use.

A number of published research reports are available in which the impact resistance of different materials has been tested according to different sizes and velocities of missiles which may be encountered.

LaMarre performed extensive experiments in the development of criteria and test methods for eye and face protective devices.[1] Wigglesworth, in two papers, compared glass, treated glass, allyl resin and polycarbonate of various thickness using missile sizes from 1/8 in. to 1 in.[2,3] Duckworth and Rosenfield compared chemically treated lenses with heat treated lenses of various thickness.[4] Kors and St. Helen reported on a massive survey of 2.2 mm ophthalmic lenses.[5] They tested untreated glass, heat treated glass, and chemically treated glass. Different ball sizes were used to obtain fractures over the range of lens materials.

Data presented by the several authors was in different terms and dimensions. Calculation and summarizing work has been done to present it in a compact format for comparison purposes.

Table 2-1 contains data from LaMarre on 3 mm thick lenses such as used in industrial safety spectacles and goggles. The average failure levels are given in terms of foot pounds energy, equivalent drop height of a 1 in. steel ball, and velocity of a 1 in. steel ball in miles per hour.

Impact energy is important as it is the only common dimension available for comparing different kinds of impact such as the drop height of a steel ball compared with the impact of a handball or a tennis ball. For some readers, drop height may be dramatic. Others may consider velocities to be more important.

While impact energy is the only common factor available for comparing many standard tests with actual accident situations, it cannot be used for comparing impacts of widely different contact areas and velocities having the same energy. For example, a 3 lb. bag of sugar dropped one foot would be unlikely to break any mounted safety lens. However, the table shows that only polycarbonate could withstand a 3 foot pound impact with a 1 in. steel ball.

Table 2-1

MEAN FRACTURE ENERGIES OF SELECTED LENS MATERIALS
INDUSTRIAL SAFETY THICKNESS (3 MM.) VARIOUS TESTS

Lens Materials	ANSI Z87.1 Requirements	Heat-Treated Glass	Allyl Resin	Polycarbonate	
1″ Steel Ball Ref. 1					
Energy Ft. Lbs.	0.62	2.1	1.3	>9.0	no failure
Equivalent drop Height (ft.)	4.2	14.0	8.7	60.0	″
Velocity MPH	11.1	20.4	16.1	42.3	″
ANSI Z87.1 Needle Test					
Penetration Velocity ft./sec.	16.3	33.7	47.3	183.0	
0.125″ Steel Ball Ref. 2, 3					
Ft. Lbs.	N.A.	0.01	0.38	4.25*	
Feet/sec.		95.0	288.0	964.0	

Author dropped 40 lb. steel plate three feet onto prescription lenses bridging 2 2 × 4″ timbers 120 ft. lbs. — No failure.

*Polycarbonate Lenses 1.9 mm. thick.

The importance of area of contact and velocity is dramatized by the 1/8 in. ball data from Wigglesworth. Except for polycarbonate, no available lens material comes close to the standard test of 0.62 foot pounds. In the standard test on average, failures do not occur until two or three times this level is obtained. It must be remembered that performance of glass lenses varies widely between samples, and some may barely pass the test.

The table also tells us why the standard glass safety lens has been so successful in many industrial situations such as construction and other areas where heavy, relatively slow-moving blows are received. Imagine a 1 in. steel ball dropped 14 ft! It also tells why there have been failures when grinding wheels fail or ricocheting bits of steel strike the lens. Small high-speed missiles are highly likely to fracture glass lenses. Plastic is far superior but not for the slower, heavy blows. Polycarbonate is the only material that can be expected to stand up to both kinds of impact. Imagine 1 in. steel balls with a velocity equivalent to a 60 ft. drop! Gas pellet guns are used to demonstrate the high-speed performance at trade shows and medical conventions. The author has experimented with lenses suspended on wires. Twenty-two caliber lead long-rifle bullets do not penetrate or break 2 mm polycarbonate prescription lenses. Twenty-two magnum shots may or may not accomplish the fracture of these lenses.

How does all of this relate to sports situations? Eye injuries in racket sports have become a critical problem. Under the auspices of the American Society for Testing Materials (ASTM) a standard setting committee has been working, and a standard for racket Sport Eye Protection has been issued (ASTM F803-85). It is currently being updated (Appendix II). The data and requirements in this standard are based on research sponsored by the committee and conducted by Professor C. R. Morehouse at Pennsylvania State University. High-speed movies were taken of actual impacts of balls and rackets on various types of eye protectors and lenses. Table 2-2 summarizes some of the data collected. Note that the velocity range and energy at impact far exceed any published impact resistance data even on polycarbonates. Even the author's steel plate test of 120 foot pounds cannot be related to velocities of 100 miles per hour.

The movies also showed that the balls sometimes deformed to a flat, bent dish. Here the impact force is spread out through time and cannot be directly related to the impact of a test steel ball. How can this situation be handled? One possibility would be to designate polycarbonate as the only hope, and cross our fingers. Fortunately, we can do better. Dr. Paul Vinger, ophthalmologist, writer, and lecturer on sports eye protection, and chairman of the ASTM Racket Sports Committee, reports that in Dr. Morehouse's study of racket sports impact, a polycarbonate lens never fractured.[12] All others have failed. Even in lensless protectors the ball deformed and penetrated the protectors. As a result of the research and the resulting Standard, properly designed products for racket sports will become increasingly available. Serious players, Racket Sport Associations, schools and colleges will expedite and enforce use of products which meet the standard. A product certification council is currently being formed.

For ice hockey, another standard (F 516-81) is being updated. This covers both open mesh and optical eye and face protectors. There is a certification council established under the auspices of the Amateur Hockey Association of the United States (Appendix II).

Participants in these structured programs will increasingly be aware of the need for effective eye protection. Unfortunately, there are many who participate in sports without the discipline and guidance which these programs provide. We see motorcyclists and bicyclists with ordinary sunglasses. Too many players in vacant lot baseball, softball, volleyball, and tennis wear ordinary sunglasses or dress prescription lenses. There is an ASTM Standard for eye and face protectors for youth baseball (Appendix II). However, when we see professional baseball and tennis players with no eye protection, it may be difficult to persuade the occasional player that he needs an expensive eye protector. Should a spontaneous game of volleyball, badminton, or softball be foregone for lack of eye protection? In such situations, especially with large balls such as the volleyball and the beach ball, the occasional risk is minimal. If sunglasses or prescription lenses are worn, they should be capable of withstanding the impact of the balls involved.

Table 2-2

BALL VELOCITY AND IMPACT ENERGY FOR CERTAIN SPORTS*

Sport	Weight (oz.)	Velocity Range (MPH)	Impact Energy (Ft. Lbs.)
Racket	1.4	85–110	21–36
Squash	0.7	130–140	25–29
Handball	2.2	55–70	14–23
Tennis	2.0	85–110	31–52

*Calculated from experimental data developed at Pennsylvania State University by Professor C. R. Morehouse for the ASTM Racket Sport Standard Committee.

Dress thickness glass and allyl resin lenses cannot be expected to withstand the input of any thrown or batted object; not even a tossed object! To prove the point, let me summarize the published data of references 2, 3, 4 and 5 for 2 mm lenses, and compare it with the energies involved in actual accidents.

For steel balls 5/8 to 1-1/8 mm in diameter—
Fracture energy in foot pounds.

	Weakest	Strongest
FDA Requires 0.15		
Glass Lenses	0.08	1.70
Allyl Resin	0.39	0.70

Polycarbonate—Not tested in these references. In house test at Gentex Corp.—no failure.

Author experiment with steel plate — 120 foot pounds.

For tests with a 1/8 in. steel ball (Reference 3) —
Average fracture energy in foot pounds.

Heat Treated Glass	1.03
Allyl Resin	0.20
Polycarbonate	4.25

It can be seen that the impact resistance of dress thickness glass or allyl resin lenses is minimal. However, eye injuries from broken spectacles in the general population are rare. Nevertheless, when the wearers are involved in sports or exposed to other risks, by intention or incidentally, accidents happen and litigation may result.

The author has been a consultant or an expert witness in several instances. Let us compare the energies involved in some of these cases with the predicted performance given above.

1. 2 mm. heat treated glass lenses were prescribed for a college baseball player. Potential impact energy 21 foot pounds. Litigation involved the prescriber, the laboratory and the *assumed* manufacturer! Recovery unknown.

2. A softball player at second base wearing sunglasses purchased at the grocery store. Maximum possible impact energy 17 foot pounds. Litigation involved the distributor and the store owner. Recovery: medical costs and lost time only.

3. Volleyball in a "dodge-em" game in school gym. Target student was not hit, but catcher wearing 2 mm glass lenses was. Minimum impact was 3 to 6 foot pounds. Allegedly, the optometrist had recommended safety glasses, but they were refused. Out of court settlement amount unknown.

4. An alcoholic beverage control officer was dropped by a haymaker swung by a bar patron. He was wearing 2 mm photochromic glasses which he had requested. Impact energy was 2 to 4 foot pounds. The contention was that his work was dangerous and that he should have been cautioned that plastic lenses were better. (Actually, plastic lenses would not have been better.) The optician was confused on the stand. The award was very large.

Other instances of eye injury from broken dress spectacles or sunglasses are listed below. Details of litigation unknown.

	Foot Pounds
Car accident, head striking dash, assume 20 mph	67.00
Flying gravel from woods bike striking rider behind	0.30–00.80
Fall, head striking corner of table	5.00–15.00
Stone thrown by lawn mower, 30 ft.	6.00–23.00
Magazine tossed across living room (assume 9 ozs. ea. ft.) (It is likely bound cover would be in the lead)	2.25

The flying gravel and stones create impacts analogous to the 1/8 in. data. The other accidents would be analogous to the drop ball data.

When the data is considered, these injuries are all predictable. The only case where allyl resin might have helped is the flying gravel from the woods bike; even that is a borderline case. Polycarbonate in sturdy frames would have prevented all of these injuries.

The lesson here is that any spectacle wearer likely to be occasionally involved in sports or other active situations, even driving, should have polycarbonate lenses. The patients' activities and interests should enter into the prescribing process. There is a need for a sports sunglass standard.

OPTICS AND VISUAL PERFORMANCE IN SPORTS

The science of testing and evaluating sports visual performance is new, developing rapidly, and controversial. It is safe to say, however, that any player will perform best if he has an accurate interpretation of his position in space and the locations of all objects of interest.

The instant a player dons an eye protector, there is not one but two worlds in which to localize. Often, each eye is presented with a different shaped world because the performance of the lenses differ between nasal and temporal viewing directions. It is also probable that some refractive error is present. This is especially true of prescription protectors.

Our sense of orientation is the result of the brain's integrating the optical and mechanical inputs with experience. High visual acuity is an asset in this process. When any lens is first worn or changed, the calibration has to be updated. Fortunately, most people adapt very quickly. What are these space distortions? First let us consider nonprescription, or "plano," eye protectors.

Plano Power Protectors

A zero power, twelve base lens will have over 1.00 prism diopters for a 30 degree angle of view, and 1.6 diopters for 40 degrees. Floors will tip down a few degrees, and peripheral fields expand. A slightly negative power has two advantages. This prism effect is reduced (but many go the other way), and a more uniform thickness lens is possible. All uniform thickness lenses have negative power. Most standards weight the power tolerance negatively. This is to accommodate any residual errors and to avoid any excess plus. Excess plus can destroy acuity, especially for driving under poor visual conditions.

The designer's goal is to achieve a balance of prismatic effects, refractive power, and adequate uniformity of thickness for safety and production purposes.

Lenses of shallower curves present less of a problem but reduce the "wrap around" effect. Several shallow curve, one piece masks have very low optical errors. The side protection is afforded by side shields or a break in the curve near the temple.

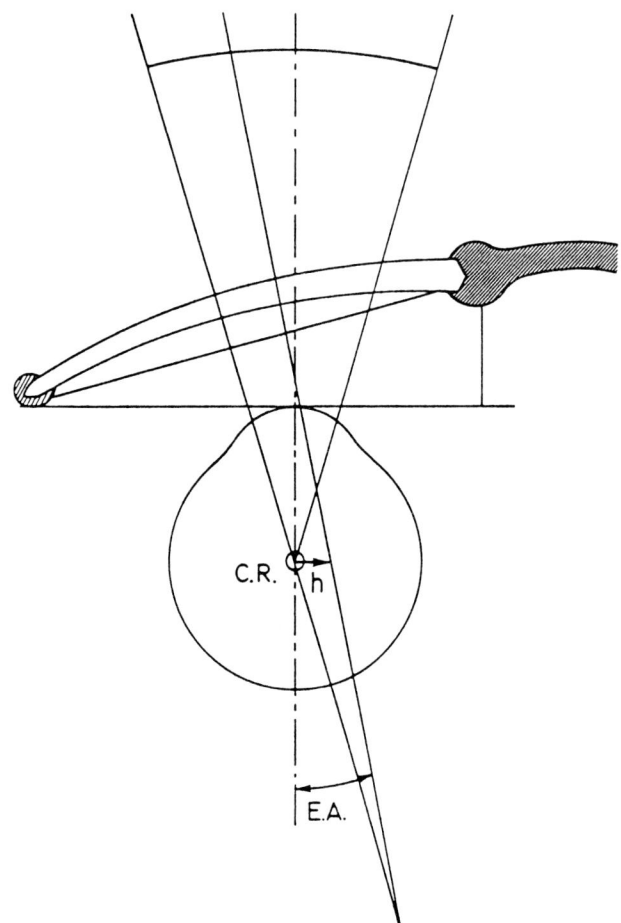

Figure 2-1. Plano or prescription lens with "Face Form" angle. Note that optical axis is decentered from the center of rotation, CR an amount of h, and is tipped an effective angle E.A. This produces prism and power imbalances especially in prescription lenses.

Some manufacturers achieve a wrap around style by angling the lenses so that optical axes of the lenses point outward (Fig. 2-1). If this face form angle exceeds 10 degrees, excess prism is introduced. There is prism imbalance between the two eyes and it varies as the eyes sweep back and forth. Wrap effect should be achieved by decentering the optical center in toward the nose, and by using as steep a curve as is necessary to achieve the desired side protection. A single lens mask has the ultimate decentration; the axis passes through the center of the nose!

The refractive properties of sports eye protection should be measured with a calibrated telescope or focimeter *as worn*, with the axis of the instrument coincident with the intended line of sight of the wearer. Table 2-3 lists the optical tolerances of pertinent standards for both plano protectors and prescription lenses.

Table 2-3

MEAN FRACTURE ENERGIES OF SELECTED LENS MATERIALS
REFRACTIVE TOLERANCES OF SELECTED STANDARDS

All Data in Diopters and Prism Diopters as Appropriate

Standard	ASTM F803-85	ASTM F513-85 draft	ANSI Z87.1-1979	ANSI Z80.1-1979	ANSI Z80.3-1977
	Racket Sports	Hockey	Industrial	Prescription	Sunglasses
Sphere or Average Power	+0.06-0.18	+0.12-0.25	+0.06	+0.13[1]	+1.125 / 0.25
Astigmatism		0.25	0.06	0.13[1]	0.125
Power Imbalance	0.18	0.25	0.12	0.26	0.18
Prism	0.50	0.50	0.06	0.33	0.25
Vertical Prism Imbalance	1.25	0.25	0.12	0.33	95% <0.50[2]
Horizontal Base In	0.25	0.25	0.12	0.66	"
Horizontal Base Out	1.00	1.00	0.12	0.66	"

[1]For lenses of +2.00 diopter. Stronger lenses have greater tolerance.
[2]Achieved by statistical quality control 95% of single lens < 0.25.
All Standards provide controls on surface waves and defects that would impair vision.

Prescription Lens Performance

The performance quality of prescription lenses has four aspects: design quality, factory quality, laboratory quality (surfacing, coating and edging), and fitting quality.

The Need for Design

As with plano lenses, the performance of a prescription lens varies with angle of view or distances of the line of sight from the optical center. Seeing postures for straight ahead viewing and minor eye excursions from one's "zero position" often involve areas of the lens 10 to 15 mm off center. In these areas, the simplest prescriptions present 0.13 diopters of sphere or cylinder error, stronger lenses present up to 0.37 diopters. These figures are the best designs. Greater errors are present if incorrect base curves are used.

Lens design consists of computing power and astigmatic errors for these off center areas. For any given vertex distance there is an ideal front base curve for each prescription. The exact choice varies slightly between designers. A good design balances the errors through an expected range of vertex distances which basically depend upon the size of the nose. For practical reasons, each base curve is used for a small range of prescriptions. The number of base curves in a series is an index of design quality.

Factory Quality

A spectacle lens is a health care product and its design should be documented and the information made available to those who prescribe or order it. For single vision lenses, a wide range of prescriptions are available from the major manufacturers in factory finished, molded uncut lenses. These are well designed multibase lens series. For prescriptions out of range and multifocals, semifinished blanks are supplied to the laboratories with charts indicating the correct blank for each prescription.

As with allyl resin and glass lenses, the number of semi-finished blanks is a function of demand. Most manufacturers supply blanks and surfacing charts that insure excellent performance for the most common prescriptions. Laboratories should follow these charts.

The surface quality can be at least as good as that of allyl resin lenses and comes close to the finest glass lenses.

The Laboratory Contribution to Quality

If the prescription is out of range of factory finished lenses or is a multifocal, it will be surfaced by the laboratory. This introduces a design decision regarding the base curve. The proper blank may not be on hand or the operator may not appreciate the importance of following the charts. In such cases, the off axis performance suffers. It is not a high quality design. There is also the question of the laboratories surfacing quality and accuracy of the finished prescription. Coating quality can be checked by visual inspection. Improper centering, edging, and mounting create prism imbalances. The quality of the final product depends on accuracy of design, proper choice of base curves and the quality of the surfacing and centering.

Fitting Quality

The off axis errors of a lens are least when its optical axis passes through or close to the sighting center of the eye. To achieve this goal, monocular interpupillary distances should be taken with a reflex pupilometer. A frame should be selected that allows for a fitting geometry similar to that of Figure 2-2. (For clarity, the side shields are not shown.) The optical axis should pass through or just below the canthus to intercept the sighting center (center of rotation) of the eye. For a 10 degree pantoscopic angle, the optical center should be about 5 mm below the

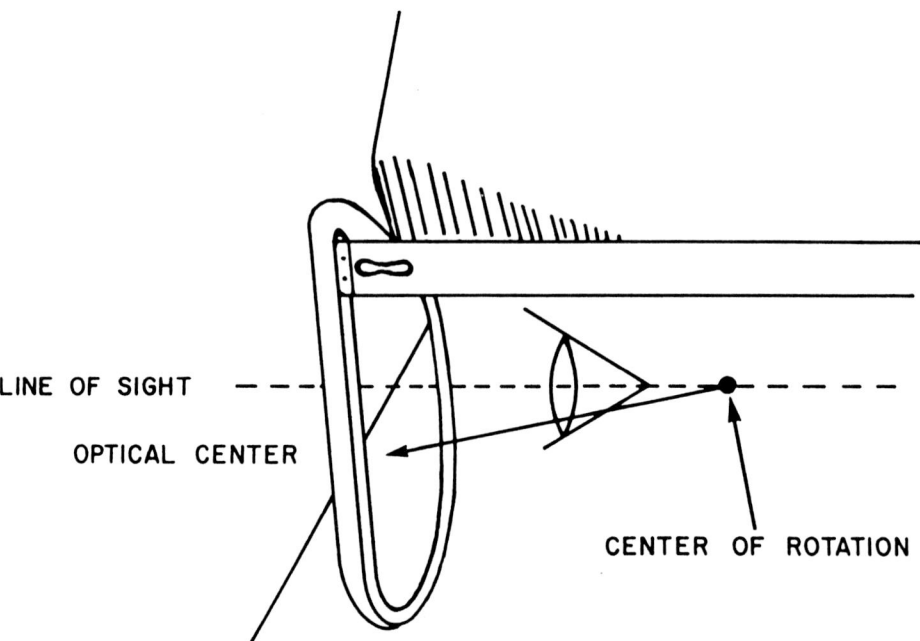

Figure 2-2. Proper vertical geometry of a prescription lens before the eye. For a 10 degree pantoscopic angle the optics center should be approximately 5 mm. below the straight ahead line of sight. Since most frames fit slightly low, the standard location of the optical center at the geometric center results in satisfactory geometry.

straight ahead line of sight as indicated by the arrow. If the lens is so fitted, it will perform as designed. Lateral angling (Face Form) as shown in Figure 2-1 introduces prism and astigmatism. It should never exceed 10 degrees and be avoided for prescriptions over ±2.00 diopters, if possible. However, there are always some patients who prefer style to optics. Sometimes mechanical considerations may take precedence.

Summary of Error Sources and Their Effects

1. Prescribing in 0.25 diopter steps. If not weighted negatively, the possible plus error can be — 0.12 diopters
2. Residual off axis errors — 0.12 to 0.37
3. Standards allow a laboratory error — 0.13 to 0.13
   Possible accumulation for full time seeing — 0.37 to 0.62
4. Face Form frame can add in one meridian — 0.10 to 0.20
   Possible accumulative total in such frames — 0.47 to 0.82
5. Face Form frames create base out prism for straight ahead seeing and imbalance as the two eyes scan right and left. Usually this is not a problem.
6. Unadapted prism — orientation problems, discomfort.
7. Minus power — probably no detriment, possibly helpful.
8. Anisometropic errors — 0.125 diopters can affect stereo and monocular acuity under critical conditions.
9. Plus power errors — a detriment to proper depth perception. For driving, street signs and freeway signs are not read in time. Allen has shown that braking distance when coming up on unlighted vehicles can be lengthened by 1 ft. per 1/100 diopter![6]

What should be done? The ophthalmologist, optometrist, or optician should have base curve charts for the lenses they order, and insist that the laboratory follow them. They should instruct the laboratory to avoid plus surfacing errors and anisometropic errors. Finally, they should select and fit frames carefully.

Absorptive Lenses

An absorptive lens controls the quantity and spectral distribution of the incident radiation. Frequently, the intensity of visible radiation, light, is reduced and the color is changed.

To some degree, every lens absorbs ultra violet and infrared radiation. When we speak of ultraviolet and infrared absorbance or transmittance, percentages are given based on the energy transmitted (watts ×

time). When we speak of the transmittance of a lens for visible radiation, we speak of *luminance transmittance,* a photometric term. Terms such as lumens, candles and foot lamberts are used to calculate and express the brightness or luminance of an object. A foot lambert or its metric equivalent expresses the brightness of a square foot of a perfectly white surface illuminated by a candle one foot away. Standard internationally accepted weighting tables are used to convert radiant energy to visible photometric terms. A watt at 450 nm has only 4 percent of the luminance of a watt at 550 nm.

The energy levels in daylight are far below retinal thresholds obtained on laboratory animals. However, there is a school of thought that blue should be differentially attenuated because of possible long-term accumulative effects. For the weekend sportsman, this concern should be negligible. For life-guards and ski instructors, brown or yellowish eye protectors would reduce any remote risk and provide more light per watt of retinal load.

THE INTELLIGENT USE OF SUNGLASSES

The ANSI Z80.3 Standard for Sunglasses and Fashion Eyewear classifies tinted lenses as follows:

Luminance transmittance greater than:

40% - Cosmetic

8-40% - General purpose attenuation of light

3 & higher* Special purpose - Ski and Boating (not driving) (Appendix II)

*special UV requirements

How these categories may be used, can be seen in Table 2-4.

Table 2-4

LUMINANCE LEVELS OF TYPICAL SCENES

Type of Scene	Luminance Foot Lamberts	Seeing Ability
Hazy sky near the sun	20,000	Glare, discomfort
Sky below the sun, sun on snow	10,000	
Whitest of beaches near white buildings	5,000	Back lighting problems
Normal beaches-light pavement	1,000-2,000	- - - - - - - - - - -
Green fields	600-1,000	
Open shade of buildings and trees	100-600	Good seeing
North facing signs on bright day	100	- - - - - - - - - - -
Deep shade	10-100	Adequate if adapted

Keeping Table 2-4 in mind, let us remember three sets of facts:

1. Average luminance greater than the 1,000 foot lamberts serves no useful purpose. Discomfort glare is likely. As scenes shift, the adaptation to lower luminances is retarded.
2. The visual grey scale from white to black is only a factor of ten. Any object that has 10 percent or less of the luminance of the surround is seen as very dark or black.
3. The instantaneous adaptive range is 2.5 to $3\times$. That is, if we are operating within a grey scale of 10-100, it can be shifted down to 3-30 or up to 30-300 while the eyes are turning to fixate one area or another.

When we face a sky luminance of 10,000 foot lamberts, highway signs and the faces of opponents in sports with a luminance of 100 foot lamberts will appear very dark and yield no information. These problems can be attenuated by wearing a cap or visor, the car sun visor or by gradient density lenses. The latter cannot help in the worst cases.

In other areas such as beaches, tennis courts and highways, the luminance levels are high but relatively uniform, especially during the middle hours of the day.

For these environments sunglasses transmitting 15 to 40 percent, will lower the entire visual environment into the "good seeing" zone without lowering the darker targets much below the 100 point, and certainly not below the 10 foot lambert level.

Patients who have prolonged exposures to large, high luminance areas such as lifeguards, ski instructors, and enthusiasts may prefer or need transmittances as low as 8 percent or less. The sunglass standard sets 8 percent as the lower limit for driving. In my opinion, patients should be cautioned about any transmittance below 12 to 15 percent.

Prescription Lens Problems

At each surface of a lens, approximately 5 percent of the incident light is reflected. As light that reaches the back surface, 5 percent is reflected forward and 5 percent of that is, again, reflected toward the eye. Figure 2-3 shows what happens in a negative lens. In a plano lens the reflected image is superimposed over the object. Since its luminance is only 0.25 percent of that of the object, no harm is done. In plus lenses, the image is pushed out in the field of view relative to the object but it is located behind the lens. For strong prescriptions, the image is located near the plane of the pupil. If bright objects are near the center of the field, this can create a veiling glare across the retina.

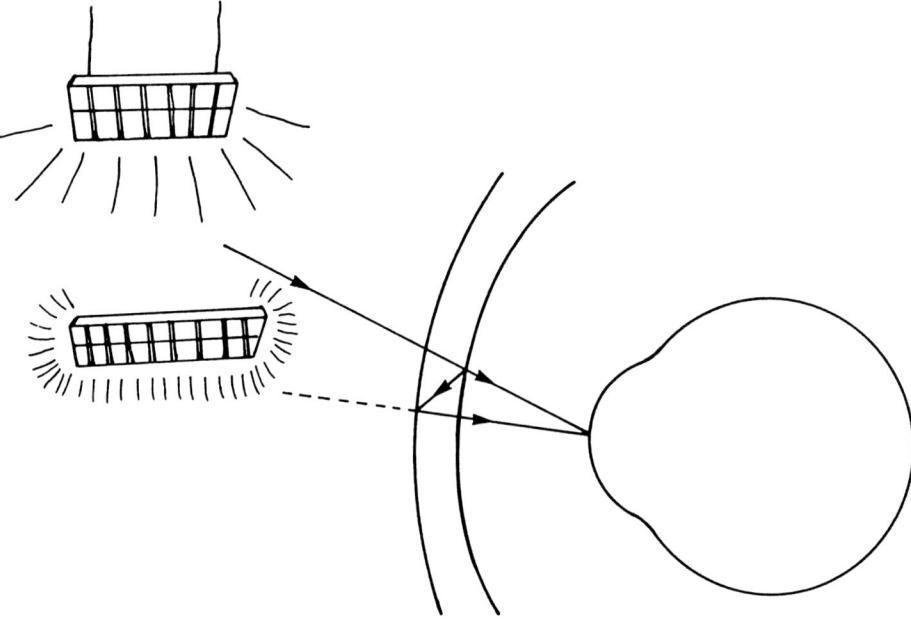

Figure 2-3. The origin of double ghost images in minus lenses. Out of doors the entire sky is lowered and reduces contrast of the entire scene, especially highway signs. Tinting attenuates the problem.

For minus lenses the reflected image of bright scenes is well defined and thrown toward the center of the field (Fig. 2-3). For driving, the bright sky is imaged over freeway signs lowering the contrast in an already difficult seeing condition. In out of door sports, the sky is imaged as a veiling glare over the opponents in the foreground.

In both cases, the problem is significant only when the sky luminance is 50 to 100 times greater than that of the foreground, as when facing the sun. Indoors, the images of lighting fixtures can be annoying.

Tinted Prescription Lenses Improve Contrast

In tinted lenses the ghost images travel the lens three times, thus greatly reducing their luminance. In a 30 percent lens, the image of the ghost will be $.30 \times .30 \times .30 = .027$, or 2.7 percent as bright as it would be in a clear lens. Even a 60 percent lens which might be acceptable for indoor sports will reduce the ghost to 22 percent of that of a clear lens, but it will not be eliminated. Even this absorption would improve contrast of back lighted signs.

Other Aids for the Prescription Wearer

Polarizing glass prescription lenses are available. If shoulder harnesses are worn, they are probably safe for driving but not for more active sports.

Polarizing flip-up clip-on lenses are a solution to the problem of rapidly changing landscapes. They can be flipped up for reading signs in the shade and going in and out of tunnels on metropolitan expressways.

Polarizing lenses are the only solution to bright specular reflections from oily pavement, car tops, and the hood of one's own car. They eliminate the image of the dash in the windshield. Some ball players might appreciate the flip-up lenses. Nonprescription formed, laminated sheet polarizing lenses are also useful for driving and general outdoor wear. They do not provide protection from racket or other sports which involve balls.

Colors of Tinted Lenses

There is little research to substantiate recommendations regarding proper colors for tinted lenses and sunglasses. The ANSI Z80.3 Sunglass Standard contains specifications for traffic signal recognition (Appendix II). The common amber and green lenses meet this requirement. The popular yellow shooting lens fails, and should not be worn for driving. Some strong amber, orange and magenta lenses suppress the green excessively.

Moderate amber and yellowish lenses yield a subjective impression of improving contrast. They do differentially darken the blue of the sky and shadows. This is useful for bird hunters and bird watchers. Skiers like them because they darken the shadows and tend to accentuate undulations in the snow. Boating enthusiasts, pilots, and control tower operators might appreciate this negative blue effect. Yellow lenses have been shown to confuse deer hunters and cause false identification. Dark blue lenses will suppress the red traffic signal. Light blue lenses are popular as a cosmetic asset. There is no evidence that they are superior for active sports or driving.

The standard green lens yields the highest luminance per watt on the retina, but it tends to shrink the width of the spectrum available to the wearer and should not be prescribed for a protanomalous patient. An amber lens might help such a patient, but would be contraindicated for the deuteranomalous.

The ophthalmologist, optometrist, or optician should be guided by the patient's interests and preferences, keeping in mind the disadvantages of the various colors. Except when darkening the sky or shadows is an advantage, neutral grey or moderate deviations from it would be indicated.

ULTRAVIOLET RADIATION

Untraviolet radiation is an increasing concern in the ophthalmic community. Figure 2-4 defines the ultraviolet spectrum, its different zones, and indicates the areas of concern. The long wave limit of ultraviolet is ambiguous. Sliney divides the spectrum as shown in Figure 2-4; UVC 100-280 nm; UVB 280-315 nm and UVA 315-400.[7] Other sources set the upper limit either at 380 or as a zone from 380-400 as shown in the figure. Analysis for color and visual transmittance starts at 380 nm. National and international standards organizations issue ultraviolet specifications up to 380 nm only, because that is where the significant, unique toxicity effects are thought to cease.

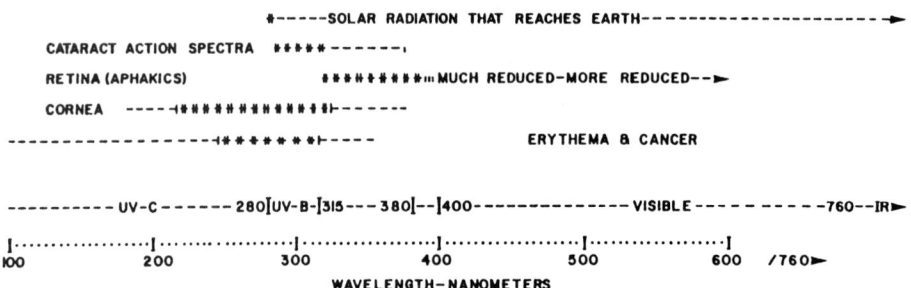

Figure 2-4. Ultraviolet and visible spectrum showing spectral regions of ocular concern; UVB 288-315 nm., UVS 315-380 nm. Retina effects extend into the visible with diminishing intensity.

UVC and UVB together contain the erythermal action spectrum including the corneal action spectrum. The upper limit is arbitrary in that the photobiological effects do not suddenly stop at a given point. Some workers set it at 315; others at 320. The UVB band describes an overlap between this upper limit and the lower limit which is the cut off point for the transmittance of the earth's atmosphere. This is now considered to be 288 nm. Therefore, current standards now define UVB as the band between 290 and 315 nm and UVA as the band between 315 and 380 nm.

The Ocular Effects of Ultraviolet Radiation

In 1981 Arthur H. Keeney, M.D., Chairman of the American National Standards Institute Ophthalmic Standards Committee Z80, appointed an *ad hoc* committee to study the effects and risks of exposure to ultraviolet radiation and to supply guidelines for writing ophthalmic lens requirements for protection (Appendix II). The members were B. Appleton, M.D.; Capt. B. R. Blais, M.D.; J. K. Davis; D. E. Eifrig, M.D.; G. A. Fry, O.D., P.H.D.; A. H. Keeney, M.D. (ex officio); W. Bickford; and D. H. Sliney, Consultant. The list included teachers and researchers in ophthalmology and optometry, military ophthalmology, and senior industrial experts in the field. The final report was presented to the parent Z80 committee in 1983. The statement on effects and risks is given below.

1. Actinic keratoconjunctivities can be induced in humans by energy having wavelength below 315 nm. Exposure of the skin's surface to actinic energy of wavelengths below 315 nm has been shown to cause the following:
   a. Erythema, sunburn
   b. Senile hyperkeratosis
   c. Basal cell carcinoma particularly of the lower lid.
   These conditions occur in susceptible individuals under actinic exposure.
2. Published action spectra for actinic keratoconjunctivitis, such as welders' flash, and snowblindness (210-315 nm) are available in reference 1 and in the ACGIH TLV Handbook (1981) (Appendix II, ref. 8).
3. Pterygium and possibly pinqueculum have long been associated with outdoor activity and sun exposure. Further, the literature implicates actinic radiation along with dehydration (low humidity) and windborne microtrauma in the cause of Climatic or Labrador Droplet Keratopathy and Spheroidal Degeneration.
4. Epidemiological data indicate that sunlight exposure and the incidence of lenticular opacities (cataracts) and possibly pseudo-exfoliation are correlated. A causal relationship has not been established. Multiple human variables such as nutritional state,

infectious disease, familial and racial genetic predisposition, and others make it difficult to assess the role played by sunlight. The waveband 295 to 320 nm has been demonstrated in the laboratory as being capable of producing lenticular opacifications in the rabbit and the primate. These laboratory data are for acute exposures, and may or may not be applicable in long-term environmental exposures. There is some deductive reasoning that long wavelength UV might play a role in the formation of cataracts. With the exception of laser exposures, the animal studies in the UVA have required high energy doses to produce damage and have not produced cataracts.
5. There is experimental evidence of retinal damage from UV radiation. There is not sufficient information to establish numerical standards for human exposure. Risk appears to increase with shorter wavelengths, aphakia, pseudophakia, photosensitizing drugs, and other variables.
6. The combined effects of ultraviolet radiation with other wavelengths have not been studied and should be evaluated. It is important to determine additive or synergistic effects of ultraviolet radiation when exposures are combined with the visible or infrared spectra.

Recommendation

It is recommended that the Standards Writing Committees require that manufacturers claiming special ultraviolet absorbing properties for their products specify the average percentage transmittance, or attenuation, of those lenses in the spectral bands 290 to 315 nm and 315 to 380 nm. Those who prescribe or recommend those products will then have adequate information.

The committee endorsed the 1977 ANSI Z80.3 Sunglass Standard noting that the requirements might not be adequate for the aphakics (Appendix II). A revision which will probably be issued in 1986 has somewhat more liberal requirements. This revision disclaims pertenance for aphakic wearers, the premise being that protection for them should be under the supervision of an ophthalmologist or optometrist.

The difficulty in writing concensus standards stems from the lack of quantitative data on accumulative effects. While Pitts has published thresholds for cataract development in rabbit eyes, cornea thresholds are much lower.[8] Development of a cataract in a few hours or even one or two days would be unlikely because the cornea would be severely damaged first.

In 1982, Ham and his colleagues reported on UVA damage to the retina of aphakic monkeys.[9] This created a new concern; the retina, and a concensus that aphakic patients need extra protection in the UVA region. As the report shows, Standards Committees have not reached agreement regarding specific requirements for protection against these unquantified, but potential long-term effects. Ultraviolet literature is extensive both with respect to laboratory and epidemiological research. Pitts, Sliney, and Parrish provide good starting points.[7,8,10] Even with the areas of controversy, the agreed upon effects are impressive. Lacking any good reason for transmitting ultraviolet, why not eliminate it?

ULTRAVIOLET IN THE ENVIRONMENT

In nonindustrial situations the principal source of ultraviolet is the sun. However, we do not look at the sun and, because of the glare, avoid postures that allow direct sunlight even obliquely to strike the eye. It is sky scatter and reflected radiation from sand and snow that are the main concerns.

The entire dome of the sky is a fairly uniform secondary source of ultraviolet with the greatest intensity in a 40 degree zone around the location of the sun. At sea level, this secondary radiation often exceeds that of the direct solar by a factor of two or more. The total radiation that reaches the ground is a function of solar height; that is, month, day, and hour. Altitude increases this total.

In early summer, in central and southern United States, UV-B on Cape Cod rivals that of the tropics. For any given time and location, the UV-B radiation is dependent on the amount of ozone, moisture, and pollutants in the atmosphere.

Light clouds and haze may increase the diffuse radiation considerably. Published data is usually for a dry, clean atmosphere, however. Thus, actual exposures are often below published data, but can also exceed it. The lighter sands reflect about 30 percent of both the direct and indirect radiation. Clear, new snow reflects about 80 percent. Water reflects very little, except certain wave forms reflect up to 20 percent and specular glistening reflections, much more.

Risks in Different Activities

The most severe sunburn is usually on the shoulders and other areas exposed to both the sun and sky when sunbathing. Most of us have had, on rare occasions, the feeling of sand in the eyes. This is a symptom of keratoconjunctivitis. The risk to the eye is a function of the *sky area* plus *ground area times reflectivity* to which the eye is exposed. The eye in its orbit is exposed to only 60 percent of the hemisphere of available radiation. For activities requiring horizontal viewing or downward viewing, the sky effect is further reduced. There the ground reflectivity becomes important. The following table gives examples of exposure times required to reach the published tolerance levels. Given times for exposure are between 11:00 A.M. and 1:00 P.M.

Spring skiing — altitude 8,500 — Colorado	30-45 minutes
Sun bathing in June — Florida	45-60 minutes
Southern New England and Central California	50-70 minutes
Golf, tennis and similar activity — same locale	2.5 hours

In February northern rates would increase four times, Florida 1.5 to two times.

Subthreshold exposures can accumulate day to day. It can be seen that the risk is greatest when exposed to large sky areas or highly reflective sand and snow areas. Concern for lesser exposures would be governed by the weight given to possible accumulative long-term effects.

Indoor Exposures

Common fluorescent lamps emit some UV-B radiation. In terms of watt per foot lambert luminance, it exceeds outdoor ratios. However, in most cases with shielded fixtures, exposure to the eye is minimal. If unshielded lamps are massed to provide high luminance, protection is advised.

Effects of Drugs

There are dramatic increases in sensitivity to ultraviolet and visible radiation induced by a variety of pharmaceutical compounds. Some examples are tetracyclines, sulfonamides, thiazides, psoralens, some oral contraceptives, and artificial sweeteners.

There should be inquiry into the patient's medication program before prescribing anything other than maximum UV protection. Because of the retinal exposure, aphakic patients should be given maximum protection to avoid solar retinitis and possible accumulative effects.

INFRARED RADIATION

Every object radiates and reflects infrared radiation. The spectrum of emission depends upon the temperature. As with the upper end of ultraviolet, the lower end of infrared is ambiguous. Most writers put it at 760 nm. However, the CIE weighting tables for visible radiation extend to 780. Thus the "IR" extends from 760-780 to about 1 nm, 1 million nm.

This very long spectrum is divided into a *near* and *far* infrared; sometimes into A, B, and C divisions as well. The near infrared is that portion transmitted by the cornea and absorbed by the aqueous, lens, and vitreous. No radiation beyond 1400 nm reaches the retina. The lens absorbs strongly between about 900 and 1400 nm. The sunglass standard defines near IR; the ACGIH tables define it as 770-1400 nm. It has generally been assumed that the cornea absorbs beyond 1400. However, some data shows transmittance into the aqueous to 2000 and beyond. Industrial standards contain requirements out to 2000 nm and beyond.

There is some concern that the iris absorbs and transfers heat to the lens. However, this aspect of concern, as well as retinal heating, is also contributed to by visible radiation. Industrial standards for retinal protection contain weighting function from 400 nm to 1400nm.

A principal concern with the heating effect of IR and visible is the probably synergistic effects which accelerate photochemical damage by ultraviolet and short-wave visible radiation. In the sports environment, however, if ultraviolet is eliminated, that problem is solved.

The principal concern for sports and other nonindustrial environments is solar at 4.5 percent, visible 45 percent, near infrared 36.5 percent and longer-wave infrared 14 percent. Early military sunglass specifications contain infrared limitations. There was no known need for this, but since the common green glasses absorbed it, there were few objections. It seemed to be a logical specification.

In addition, the *glass blowers cataract* was understood to be the result of infrared radiation. The manufacturers of green glass sunglasses were happy to let it stand and made the most of it. As plastic lenses came into use, the need was reevaluated. It is more difficult to provide near IR absorbance in either allyl resin or polycarbonate lenses. Their advantage is weight and current national and international sunglass standards do not require IR absorbance.

CUMULATIVE EFFECTS

A dominant concern with ultraviolet is long-term accumulative photochemical effects of subthreshold exposures, because these effects have been shown to accumulate in the short term. In all experiments the damage by long-wave visible and infrared is mainly thermal. Photochemical effects in the infrared are estimated only and, therefore, are doubtful. In the ACGIH guidelines the weighting function is 1/1000 of the thermal function (Appendix II). There is no evidence that subthreshold thermal effects are cumulative. If they were we would destroy our cornea and retina after a few evenings before the fireplace.

Glass Blowers Cataract

Pitts and Cullen analyzed the original literature that supported the existence of this phenomenon.[11] They found that when the radiant source and filters (water) were identified, the incident radiation had to be ultraviolet, not infrared.

In the same paper, they also reported on production of *temporary* cataracts with near infrared radiation. The energy required was 4000 to 6000 joules (watt seconds).

Infrared Exposures

Where in nonindustrial situations might such exposures occur? How do they relate to the ACGIH guidelines for "possible delayed effects upon the lens of the eye or cataractogenesis"? (Appendix II) These guidelines suggest 0.01 watts per square cm as a limit. The sky has negligible near infrared. The direct solar radiation normal to the sun is quite uniform throughout the year. Grass and foliage reflect 20 to 30 percent, buildings and sand reflect much less. The main concern, again, is fresh snow which reflects 75 percent. Gazing at a level field of snow with no sky or trees in view, an observer would just attain the ACGIH limit of 0.01 watts/cm^2. If the view were half sky, the exposure would be halved. (See Table 2-4.) At 0.01 watts/cm^2 it would take 111 hours without changing posture or blinking to attain the Pitts and Cullen temporary cataract threshold.

We can conclude that infrared is not an ocular problem in the sports environment, with one exception. Sitting before the fire, after a day of skiing, the incident near infrared may be more than twice the ACGIH guidelines. However, there is little visible and no ultraviolet to give any concern with synergistic effects. An amateur blacksmith suffered frequent injection and discomfort. Light green IR absorbing lenses solved the problem. Those who operate barbeque pits might appreciate IR protection as well.

MATCHING PRODUCTS TO THE NEEDS

We have discussed the needs for quality lens performance and the origin of those needs. Let us now compare and summarize how well the different products meet those needs.

Lens Materials Compared

For protection against mechanical risk there is but one candidate, polycarbonate. For plano lenses and factory molded single vision prescription lenses, a 2 mm. thickness is adequate. However, the ANSI Z87.1 standard requires 3 mm. thickness for separate lenses in a frame (Appendix II).

For driving with seat belts and other activity where mechanical risk is not the dominant concern, there are other candidates. The different materials are compared below.

Weight, Thickness and Index Factors

	Glass	*Allyl Resin*	*Polycarbonate*
Center Thickness (mm)	04.60	04.73	04.30
Weight in grams	23.60	12.50	10.70

Minus lenses would have a similar relationship for edge thickness and weight.

Refractive Index	1.523	1.498	1.586
Dispersion (NU Value)	58.00	58.00	30.00
Specific Gravity	02.53	01.81	01.20
Visual Transmittance	92.%	92.%	92.%
			with coatings

The combination of high index and low specific gravity makes polycarbonate the lightest and thinnest lens available. For example: +3.00 diopter lens, 60 mm. round, 2mm. edge.

Table 2-5

PROPERTIES AND PRODUCT TYPES OF POPULAR LENS MATERIALS

Properties	Poly-carbonate	Coated Allyl Resin	CR-39	Glass
Safety	1	3*	2-3*	2-3*[1]
Weight	1	2	2	3
Thickness	1	2	2	2-3
Optics	Can be equal, depends on availability of base curve			
Abrasion Resistance	2	2	3	1
Ghost Image Reduction	1	1	2	3[2]
U. V. Blocking	1	1-2**	1-2**	3***
Semi-Finished Blanks				
Single Vision	1	1	1	1
Bifocals	1	1	1	1
Trifocals	1	1	1	1
Progressives	-	1	1	1
Laboratory Coatings	1	1	1	-
Laboratory Tinted Coatings	1	1	1	-
Photochromics	-	2	2	1
Polarized Lenses	?F	F	PFR	PFR
Bulk and/or Dyed Tints	P?	PR	PR	PR
Gradient Density	P	PR	PR	R (vacuum film)
One Piece Eye Protectors	P	P	P	(also other sheet plastic)

*Relative impact resistance depends on type of missile.
**Different degrees of UV absorbance are available.
***Depends on product and density of color, no true blocking to 380 nm.

1. Corning supplies a polyurethane backed lens — much safer than ordinary glass. Not recommended for active sports.
2. Vacuum deposited antireflection film is effective.

P = Plano
R = Rx
F = Flip up available
? = May become available

Dispersion, NU value 30: As with any high index material, the NU value is lower than for low index materials. This results in an increase in lateral chromatic aberration. Discerning patients may notice colored fringes along black edged borders and letters at wide field angles with lenses of over 2.00 diopters. For lenses 5.00 diopters and more, there have been a few comments received. For such patients, lenses of a different material might possibly be preferred for passive outdoor wear. The trade-offs between weight, safety, and edge of field color could be discussed especially if the patient participates in sports. Polycarbonate should not be used for cataract spectacles. It is top choice for use with intraocular implants.

Problems with Polycarbonate

There are occasional black specks and coating specks as with all coated lenses, and sometimes coating marks around bifocal segments. The criteria for acceptance is that used in the military; is it visible to the wearer in the *as worn* position?

1. Chemical Attack: Coated lenses are inert to most solvents. The uncoated edge can be attacked. Care should be exercised against carbon tetrachloride.
2. Need for Care: Improper edging, improper surfacing, and too heavy or poorly applied coatings can weaken polycarbonate as they will allyl resin lenses. Instructions should be followed and help obtained if there are problems.
3. Availability: Uncut finished single vision lenses in both 2 mm. and 3 mm. thickness are available over a wide range of prescriptions, and the range is increasing. Table 2-4 lists and ranks the various materials with respect to their properties and lens type availability. The technology of molding, dying, tinting, and of adhesives for films is rapidly developing. New and improved products are continuously being developed.

The racketball eye protectors provide the maximum safety in eye wear. However, not everyone wants or needs or would wear such products for all purposes. There is a place for other levels of performance.

Levels of Performance and Protection of Sports Eyewear

At all levels the refractive and absorptive performance should add to the visual performance, if possible, and inherent decremental features should be minimized.

Level 1

Products designed and advertised for particular sports should protect against the mechanical and radiation risks of the designated sport. The wearer should be at less risk with the product than without it. A list of current standards for specific sports is given in Appendix II.

Professionals and serious amateurs who regularly participate in particular sports should have Level 1 products if available.

Level 2

General purpose *sports* sunglasses and prescription spectacles clear, or tinted. These should be of materials and design so that in a sports activity the wearer is not at greater risk than without them. Children, and all who may participate in a softball, volleyball, or vacant lot baseball, and may not afford or want special products, should have this level. Even in this level, differences in design can be selected for various purposes. For example, for mountaineering or occasional skiing, wrap around lenses will give better UV protection.

Level 3

Products where special features or dress style requirements outweigh mechanical and radiation protection concerns. Examples of such products are photochromic and polarizing lenses, general purpose sunglasses, where style or cost consideration are dominant. These products may well be an asset in driving (with seat belts fastened) and be satisfactory for passive beach wear. Sunglasses should meet the ANSI Z80.3 Standard (Appendix II). Patients should be warned that there are safer products.

SPORTS SUNGLASSES AND SPECTACLES DEFINED

Vinger states a need for a sports sunglass standard.[12] With his help the following definition of a sports sunglass or spectacle is presented.

Definition

A sports sunglass or spectacle that creates no risk for the wearer and is capable of providing all benefits implied by its appearance and construction.

Requirements:

1. Size and shape should be such that in frontal impact the assembly will be supported by the bone structure around the eye to protect the eye from contact by the lens.

2. The frame shall be of a material and construction that will not fracture under the impact of baseballs, softballs, and the like.
3. The frame shall have a lens retaining lip as required by ANSI Z87.1979.
4. The temples shall be blocked from opening beyond 90 degrees.
5. The lenses shall be polycarbonate.
6. The lenses shall meet all the requirements of ANSI Z80.3 pertinent to the level of transmittance and any special features such as polarization or gradient density.
7. The lenses shall transmit less than 1 percent of UVB and UVA from 290 to 380 nm.
8. If the color or transmittance does not meet the requirements of ANSI Z80.3 for driving, the product shall be so labeled.

Other Dispensing Considerations

There are attractive frames that meet the safety requirements of ANSI Z87 but that may fracture when struck by a racketball. These may not be large enough for the *sports* Level 2 designation, but are adequate for the *do-it-yourself* hobbyist. They are also safer than dress frames for accidents of any kind. These should be considered in Level 3 situations.

EQUIPPING ONESELF AND DECISION MAKING

Appendix I contains a matching of available special products with recommended uses. Research is going on in a number of sports which will lead to products and standards for those sports. For the busy ophthalmologist, optometrist, or optician, keeping up can be a problem. However *sports vision* is really another expression for top quality visual performance and safety. Everyone is entitled to that. An assistant can be delegated to scan all advertising, exhibit literature, journal articles, and direct mail for new products or changes in products. They can write to manufacturers requesting specific information on materials, optical design, and ultraviolet transmittance for all the products of interest. Each year the *Optical Index* publishes "Dispensers Source Book" (Professional Press). This lists all manufacturers and their products. It is a good issue to keep.

Many ophthalmologists are reluctant to prescribe more than one pair of glasses. We do not wear the same clothes for different activities. In addition to any sports spectacles such as racket sports or hunting glasses, glasses for driving and the home shop might well be different than those for the office or social affairs. Top quality shoes and jackets share about the same cost as spectacles. If we have three pairs of shoes, why not three pairs of spectacles?

While polycarbonate is the only material that should be considered for notched and drilled mounting, such mountings should not be used for any sports use, even driving. Neither should frames with adjustable pads that could penetrate the eye on impact.

Lastly, aphakics with intraocular implants or contact lenses may need complete ultraviolet protection. One-eyed patients need polycarbonate lenses and the maximum practical safety in a frame.

APPENDIX I

List of Recommended Applications by Product Type

Racket Sports Eye Protection

Racket sports, soccer, baseball (research is going on regarding these two), basketball, first choice for softball, second choice for street and floor hockey. Football under face guards.

Eye and Face Protectors for Hockey Players

Ice hockey, street and floor hockey.

Motorcycle Goggles, Face Masks (NSC-8)

Motorcycling and snowmobiling. Optics of the standard cannot be met but standard should be used for mechanical features.

Youth Baseball Face Protectors

Youth baseball and softball.

Alpine Skiers' Eye Protectors

Skiers, snowmobiling (second choice)

Swimming, Diving Goggles

Swimming, diving; goggles should have no sharp edges, not too tight and polycarbonate lenses.

Diving Masks

Snorkel and scuba diving. Masks vary in thickness and safety. The better ones are at least 5 mm. thick. Prescription lenses with flat fronts can be bonded to the inside surface.

Sports Sunglasses and Spectacles (Our Level 2)

Softball (second choice), volleyball, running, mountaineering and sailing (with side protectors for UV), horseback riding, cycling, skeet, bird, and BB shooting (steep wrap or side shields) game hunting (presbyopic shooter should have bifocal segment in and high, fitted by experiment with actual gun). Yellow not recommended for game hunting. Driving (see discussion). All general wear where other considerations do not take precedence. Patient should be cautioned whenever Level 3 products are prescribed. Photochromics and nonpolycarbonate polarizing lenses are examples.

Polycarbonate Lenses in Patients' Choice of Frame

All other activities unless some positive reason for contraindication. The sturdier the frame the better.

APPENDIX II

Selected Available Standards

Pertinent to Sports Eye Protection
American Society for Testing Materials, Inc. (ASTM)
1916 Race Street
Philadelphia, Pa. 19103

Qualifications for faceguards for youth baseball ASTM F910.

Eye protection for use by players of racket sports, standard specification F803-85, 1983. (Revised 1985).

Eye and face protective equipment for hockey players ASTM F513-81 (Revision underway 1985).

Alpine Skiers — Specifications for Eye Protective Devices ASTM F659.

Canadian Standards Association (CSA)
178 Rexdale Boulevard
Rexdale (Toronto), Ontario, Canada
MSW 1R3

Face protectors for ice hockey and box lacrosse players. Canadian Standards Association, National Standard of Canada.

Racket Sports eye protection, preliminary standard P400-M 1942, CSA.

Industrial eye and face protectors CSA Z94.3 — M1982.

American National Standards Institute, Inc. (ANSI)
1430 Broadway
New York, N.Y. 10018

American National Standard Practice for occupational and educational eye and face protection. ANSI Z87.1, 1979.

American National Standard Requirement for first quality prescription ophthalmic lenses ANSI Z80.1, 1979.

American National Standard Requirements for nonprescription sunglasses and fashion eyewear ANSI Z80.3, 1977.

Vehicle Equipment Safety Commission
Suite 802, 4660 Kenmore Avenue
Alexandria, Virginia 22304

Minimum requirements for motorcyclists eye protection. VESC-8, 1980.

ACGIH, American Conference of Governmental Industrial Hygenists
6500 Glenway Avenue
Building D-5
Cincinnati, Ohio 45211

(For ultraviolet and blue exposure limits) TLVSR threshold limit values for chemical substances in workroom air adapted by ACGIH for 1980 (revisions periodically).

Amateur Hockey Association of the United States
2997 Broadmoor Valley Road
Colorado Springs, Colorado 80906

REFERENCES

1. LaMarre, David A.: *Development of Criteria and Test Methods for Eye and Face Protective Devices.* NIOSH Research Project, U.S. Dept. of Health, Education and Welfare Public Health Service, Center for Disease Control, National Institute for Occupational Safety and Health, Contract No. 210-75-0058, Aug. 1977.
2. Wigglesworth, E.C.: The impact resistance of eye protector lens materials. *Am J Optom, 48:* 245, 1971.
3. Wigglesworth, E.C.: A comparative assessment of eye protective devices and a proposed system of acceptance and grading. *Am J Opt, 49:* 287, 1972.
4. Duckworth, W.H., and Rosenfield, A.R.: Strength of thin chemtempered lenses: drop ball testing. *Am J Optom Physiol Opt, 5:* 801, 1978.
5. Kors, Kermit, and St. Helen, Roger: Base line fracture resistance studies of tempered and non-tempered glass ophthalmic lenses. *Am J Opt, 50:* 632, 1973.
6. Allen, Merril J.: *Vision and Highway Safety.* Philadelphia, Chilton, 1970.
7. Sliney, David, and Wolbarsht, Myron: *Safety with Lasers and Other Optical Sources: A Comprehensive Handbook.* New York, Plenum, 1980.
8. Pitts, D.G.: The ocular effects of ultraviolet radiation. *Am J Optom Physiol Opt, 55:* 19, 1978.
9. Ham, W.T., Jr., Mueller, H.A., Ruffolo, J.J., Jr., Guerry, D., III, and Guerry, R.K.: Action spectrum for retinal injury from near-ultraviolet radiation in the aphakic monkey. *Am J Ophthalmol, 96:* 299, 1982.
10. Parrish, J.A., Anderson, R.R., Urbach, R., and Pitts, D.G.: *Biological Effects of Ultraviolet Radiation with Emphasis on Human Response to Longwave Ultraviolet.* New York, Plenum, 1978.
11. Pitts, D.G., and Cullen, A.P.: Determination of infrared radiation levels for acute ocular cataractogenesis. *Graefes Arch Clin Exp Ophthalmol, 217:* 285, 1981.
12. Vinger, Paul F.: The eye and sports medicine. In Duane, Thomas D.: *Clinical Ophthalmology.* Philadelphia, Harper & Row, 1985.

CHAPTER 3

COLOR VISION

Cynthia MacKay

WHAT CAUSES objects to have color? Basically, it is because all objects absorb certain wave lengths of light and reflect others. Red objects are red because they reflect red light and absorb all other colors. Green plants will flourish under a red light, which their green chlorophyll absorbs well, but will die under a green light, which they reflect. Black objects absorb all the light that strikes them, while white objects reflect all the light. Therefore, a white shirt is to be preferred over a black one for sports wear on a hot sunny day. A dark colored or black jacket is better for winter sports.

What is the purpose of color vision? Wouldn't we get around just as well if we saw the world only in white and black? The answer is that color vision enables us to distinguish an object from its background. If our eyes saw only black and white, we could only pick out an object if it was whiter (brighter) or blacker (darker) than its background. However, if we also used color as a clue, we could see an object against a background even if it was of the same brightness, providing it was of a different color. For example, it is much easier to recognize and avoid shooting a fellow hunter if he is dressed in red or orange rather than in brown or green.

The human eye is a combination of a daytime eye (composed of receptors called cones), and a nighttime eye (made up of receptors called rods). It is the cones, not the rods, that are able to see color. The cones act when there is bright light entering the eye, but they are not active in dim light. The rods, in contrast, are bleached out in daylight but come into play when the light fades; therefore, we see only black and white at night. Humans have good all purpose eyes which function over an amazingly wide range of illumination. This is not true of all animals. Rats, for example, have only rods in their eyes and therefore are "day blind." Conversely, ground squirrels have only cones in their eyes and are "night blind."

Three different kinds of cones are needed for normal color perception: red cones, blue cones, and green cones. If all three cones are present and functioning normally, a person has normal trichromatic (three color) vision. If either the red cones or the green cones are not functioning, or are functioning weakly, a person will have red-green color blindness. If the blue cones are defective, a person will have blue-yellow color blindness. Such people have dichromatic (two color) vision.

Not many animals are trichromatic. Dogs and cats are dichromatic. Bulls are also dichromatic and are red-green color blind; they cannot tell the difference between red, green, or yellow. Presumably, matadors selected the red cape color to appeal to the ladies in the balcony rather than to attract the bull. Certain birds of prey are tetrachromatic: they have four different cones and must, therefore, see colors that humans cannot. What these colors look like, we can only guess.

Very few people, perhaps one in 100 million, have only one type of functioning cones in their eyes. These people are called "cone monochromats." They see the world in shades of black and white only.

Red-green color blindness is caused by a recessive gene on the X chromosome. Genes carried on the X chromosome are called sex-linked or X-linked. Women have two X chromosomes, while men have an X and a Y. Therefore, red-green color blindness is much more common in men than in women. A woman who inherits a bad X chromosome from one parent will almost always have a healthy X from the other parent to compensate for it, but a man who inherits a faulty X will always have the disease.

Roughly nine percent of males have some type of a red-green color blindness (18 million men in the United States alone), while only 0.5 percent of women are color defective. This means that almost one out of every ten men will have some difficulty in distinguishing red from green. Many men are so mildly affected that they are unaware of the problem, until they are tested.

Women transmit color blindness, but rarely suffer from it. A woman who carries a defective X chromosome will, on the average, pass it on to half of her sons. Men suffer from color blindness, but do not transmit it.

Since a boy receives only his Y chromosome from his father, he cannot inherit his father's color blindness.

Color blindness prevents people from holding certain jobs, for instance, airline or ships' pilots and railroad engineers. In certain states they cannot be policemen. Obviously, they do not do well as interior decorators or painters. A red-green color blind football player would have difficulty recognizing his team mates if they had red uniforms and the opposing team had green uniforms. On the contrary, color blindness is considered to be an asset in military intelligence. Men who completely lack green cone function, the so-called deuteranopes, are very insensitive to camouflage and can be used to detect enemy installations in color photographs. By using brightness cues instead of color cues, they can pick up a slight difference of intensity between camouflage and natural background.

There are several tests for color blindness which have varying degrees of specificity and sensitivity. An inexpensive but sensitive test which is widely used is the Ishihara plates, composed of red or green numbers on a green or red background. This test is good in that it will pick up very mild red-green color problems, but it has a few disadvantages. Primarily, in order to use this test, the patient must know numbers. Secondly, this test does not detect blue-yellow color blindness and, finally, this test does not judge the severity of the red-green deficiency. Slightly more expensive, the Farnsworth Panel d-15 is a series of fifteen colored discs that are arranged in order, by the patient. It is easy for all ages to use, even small children. In addition, this test will detect both blue-yellow and red-green color problems. However, it does miss very mild color deficiencies. The best color test ever devised, the AOHRR plates, is unfortunately no longer manufactured.

It is possible to acquire color blindness even if you are not born with the problem. Certain drugs can cause either temporary or permanent color blindness. Some of the drugs taken for tuberculosis, especially INH® and Ethambutol,® can gradually cause red-green color blindness if taken for an extended time period. The same is true of the antibiotic, Chloramphenicol.® People who are taking Digoxin® (or Lanoxin®) will start to experience blue-yellow color blindness if they are taking too much of this drug; indeed, this is a convenient early warning symptom of an overdose.

If you start to develop a cataract, you will often acquire blue-yellow color blindness because the lens turns a yellow-brown as it ages, and screens out blue light. After cataract surgery, you will again see blues in all of their brilliance.

Patients with macular degeneration will acquire red-green color blindness if the condition becomes severe enough to destroy most of their central vision. Conversely, patients with severe end-stage glaucoma, will develop blue-yellow color blindness, once their peripheral vision is destroyed.

People who smoke and drink very heavily and eat poorly may develop red-green color blindness. Fortunately, they can gain back their color perception by cutting down on the cigarettes and alcohol, taking vitamins, and eating more fresh fruits and vegetables.

People who suffer from multiple sclerosis will very commonly have inflammation of the optic nerves. The nerve usually recovers, but the patient will often be left with some mild color deficiency, even though the central vision is normal.

What is the ideal color for the ball in racquet sports? There are several different factors to take into account before making that decision. First, you would want a ball that will contrast with the background. The background will vary, of course, with different sports. In outdoor sports, such as baseball and tennis, the ball must stand out against the blue and/or white sky. It must also be visible against the ground, which is green and/or brown. Blue, green and brown would be poor color choices for these sports. White, which is actually a mixture of all colors, more than makes up for its contrast deficiencies due to its greater brightness or luminence. In squash, which is played in a white court, the best ball color is black although a very dark green ball is also often used.

Secondly, when selecting a ball for a given sport, you will want to choose one that will appear very bright to the human eye. The retina is most sensitive to yellow, so this is always a good choice for a ball color. Reds and blues are not strong stimulants to the retina, so these colors are less desirable.

In the third place, you will not want to use a red or green ball for a given sport, as nine percent of all men are red-green color defective. Such men cannot find a red croquet ball in a field of green grass because to them, both red and green have the same color value.

Ophthalmologists are often asked, "What is the ideal color for sunglasses which are to be used in sports?" The best all purpose color is a neutral gray because it will not distort color perception in any way. The lenses should be dark enough so it is difficult to see the wearer's eyes through them. Fishermen often use yellow-tinted glasses, because the yellow pigment absorbs blue light which is very highly scattered because of its short wave length. The glare off the surface of a rippled stream is largely composed of blue light. When this light is absorbed, the fish underneath stand out very clearly.

Glare also becomes a problem when driving or playing sports at dusk. When you do not want to use a darkly-tinted lens, a good way to solve this particular problem is to use polarized glasses. Glare tolerance decreases with increasing age, with the development of cataracts, with diabetics who have suffered bleeding in the eye, and with people who wear contact lenses. Such people should also use polarized lenses while driving or playing sports in glare conditions.

At present, there is no known treatment for color blindness. A patient can improve his performance on standard color tests by wearing a colored filter or a red-tinted contact lens in one eye only. The filter enhances brightness contrasts; red dots stay red while green dots become darker. However, this is a far cry from normal color vision. In addition, use of a red lens may actually be dangerous if worn while playing sports, as it darkens vision and distorts depth perception.

In conclusion, the essence of the problem of color blindness in sports is that some patients, playing certain sports, may be able to adjust and play quite normally. Others, depending on their particular type of color blindness and the circumstances surrounding the sport, may never be able to participate successfully.

CHAPTER 4

FOOTBALL

Eugene M. Helveston

THE STANDARD visual requirements for playing football will vary according to the position played, the level of football competition, and the unique requirements and/or wishes of the individual. So-called skill positions, or those which require handling of the football by either passing, receiving, receiving handoffs, fielding punts, or kicking field goals or extra points, require good visual acuity including good depth perception. Other positions such as interior linemen, tackle, guard, some special teams' members (kick-off, returns etc.), and offensive center, except for when long center passes are required for punts and place kicks, can be played adequately with some reduction in visual acuity and/or binocular functioning. The potential risk for eye injury, on the other hand, is about of equal magnitude. Any position on the football team places the eye more or less in equal jeopardy with regard to injury from a variety of causes.

Little apparent variation in ideal visual capability or concern regarding potential injury exists between junior organized football and higher levels up through the sport played at the professional level. That is, it is advantageous to have normal acuity and stereopsis at skill positions regardless of the competitive level of activity in the sport and all appropriate steps should be taken to avoid injury. However, since playing on a recreational basis may require less excellence in all areas as compared to playing on a professional basis, actual visual requirements may play a less significant role. Most of the experiences that I relate here deal with what I have learned as an ophthalmology consultant to a professional football team. While differences exist, there is certainly less variation in the *eye* health of football players at all levels than there is in the area of football skills and intensity of play. That is, football players' eyes are more alike than football players' skills.

Eye care, as is the case with most health needs of the professional football player, is carried out in a more exhaustive manner than they are at lower levels of organized football. However, most aspects of visual function and the need for care are probably the same or at least similar. The coaching staff and medical support personnel at any level of organized football should be concerned that the best interest regarding ocular health of all of their players is maintained. In this regard, all organized football might attempt to emulate the example of the professional football ophthalmic program. As an addition to purely health considerations in the case of the professional athlete, the eye health program also deals with legal and contractual requirements related to the player's personal well-being and disability factors associated with financial responsibility related to any injury. In the case of the professional athlete or the athlete sponsored by a college or high school, it is important to be fully aware of any preexisting ocular health factors so that they may be differentiated from acute or current problems.

THE EYE EXAMINATION FOR THE FOOTBALL PLAYER

A physical examination carried out by the ophthalmologist should establish several baseline criteria and accomplish the following:

1. Determine the state of ocular health as a part of the general physical examination. This is particularly useful in establishing whether some loss of visual function is new and related to a current injury or whether it was preexisting. The longer an individual is involved in a given sport, the more likely it is that some type of problem may exist. For example, I have made the observation that athletes from a sunny climate often have chronically inflamed pinguecula or pterygia. The incidence of pterygium in professional football players appears to be higher than that of the population as a whole.
2. The eye examination should uncover treatable ocular conditions that may be found in any type of a routine examination.
3. The general physical examination should insure that the minimum criteria for eligibility to play are met. These criteria can be arbitrarily established.

EYE EXAMINATION AND PROGRESS REPORT
INDIANAPOLIS COLTS FOOTBALL

NAME_____ POSITION_____

AGE____ / ___ / _____

HISTORY

GLASSES: YES   NO   CONTACTS: YES   NO

OD   SPH   CY   AX   OD

OS   OS

RNS   SPH   CY   AX   TA

OD   OD

OS   OS

VISION   DIST   W/O GLASSES   NEAR   STEREO   FLY   ABC   9/

OD   20/   20/   J#

OS   20/   20/   J#

                                              COLOR

MOTILITY   PCT

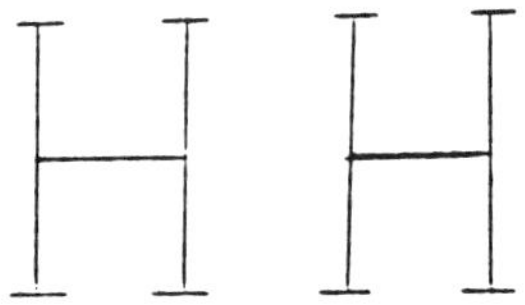

                                  NPC

EXT   XL: NORMAL   OTHER
                                  CORNEA   _____   _____
                                  AC   _____   _____
                                  LENS   _____   _____
                                  IRIS   _____   _____

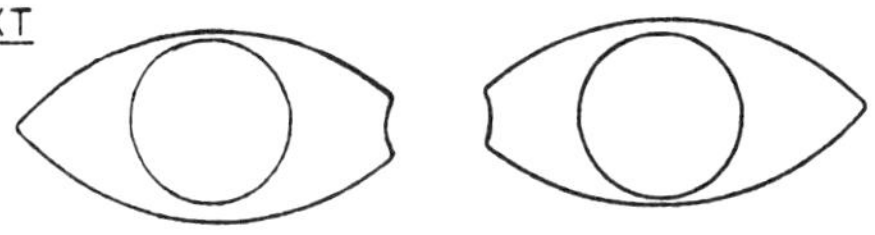

FUNDUS

COMMENT:_____

Figure 4-1. Form used for the eye examination for the Indianapolis Colt's Football Team.

A simple form used for physical examination of the Indianapolis Colt's Football Team is included (Fig. 4-1). Visual functions that are checked include visual acuity both at distance and near, with and without correction, either with spectacles or contact lenses. Stereo acuity is examined using the Titmus test. Manifest refraction is carried out if visual acuity is less than 20/20 each eye at distance. This is, in nearly every case, followed up by a full in-office examination which includes cycloplegic refraction and postcycloplegic acceptance for prescription of an optical correction. Color vision is tested with the AOHRR (or equivalent) color plates. Confrontation visual fields are carried out testing each eye. Versions (binocular ocular rotations) are tested in the eight diagnostic positions. Ductions (monocular eye movements) are also carried out in the eight diagnostic positions. Cover testing to determine the presence or absence of a latent or manifest strabismus or eye crossing is carried out at the distance in straight ahead gaze and also at near. Intraocular pressure is determined with a Schiotz or air-puff tonometer. Fundus examination is carried out through the undilated pupil. Observation of the anterior segment of the eye is done with a biomicroscope. Pupillary reactions are tested directly and consensually with a pen light.

An ocular history is obtained which includes direct questioning regarding the use of eye medicines, prior eye surgery, glaucoma in the family, or any previous injuries or other eye problems.

REFRACTIVE ERROR

About 20 percent of professional football players need some type of optical treatment for nearsightedness, farsightedness, astigmatism or a combination of these. I would expect that a similar statistic would be present for players at the college and high school level according to experience gained in treating children, adolescents, and young adults. In about 90 percent of these cases this refractive error (need for optical correction) is treated with the use of contact lenses. Contact lenses for use while playing football may be the so-called "hard" daily wear type or they may be one of a variety of "soft" oxygen permeable, extended wear types. However, even when using extended wear types of contact lenses, we prefer that these be worn on a daily basis with removal for cleaning and storage at night. In order to make this realistic, it is appropriate for an athlete to have the slightly more rigid oxygen permeable lenses compared to the thin "floppy" type. The typical small diameter, fairly steep fit, daily wear hard lenses are more prone to pop out with contact and are generally not preferred by athletes in contact sports. Hard lenses have excellent optical characteristics, they produce good vision, are less expensive and more durable, and are easier to clean. However, the fact that they are frequently lost makes them less than ideal for the football player. However, if hard contact lenses are worn, it is a good practice to have one or more complete sets available for a back-up. Fortunately, the days of holding up nationally televised sporting events while a contact lens is being searched for appear to be over. There is a tendency now among football players and other athletes toward wearing the larger, soft, oxygen permeable contact lenses. Modern contact lenses have better fit characteristics, are more comfortable, and stay on the eye far better than the early soft lenses. However, it is only fair to say that while soft lenses are more comfortable and stay on the eye better, they may offer slightly inferior optical characteristics, are harder to clean, are more fragile, and can at times lead to corneal vascularization. The professional athlete should have one or more back-up contact lenses available, but this may not be feasible for the recreational athlete. However, the implications of a lost contact lens will also not be the same for the recreational player as it could for the professional who, on the basis of performance on a single play, has to worry about the consequences which may be as serious as missing the league championship or even the Superbowl.

About 10 percent of football players at the professional level who require optical correction have this treated with spectacles. When spectacles are worn by the football player, they should be of the special, sport type variety. "Rec Specs", for example, are a very suitable athletic frame (Fig. 4-2). These glasses are shown in the illustration. Soft nose padding covers a broad area over the bridge of the nose and forehead and side temple padding helps to absorb lateral shocks. A straight, broad temple piece with a strap that goes around the back of the head ensures a secure fit for the glasses frame. The lenses are made from polycarbonate material which provides safety in that this type of lens material will not break or shatter even after tremendous impact. The lenses are also placed securely into the frame so they will not pop out or dislocate on contact.

The use of suitable face protection attached to the football helmet in the form of a face guard provides additional protection for the player's face and for the spectacles when they are worn. The spectacle lenses can be tinted if needed. Several of our players selected a light blue tint. This did not prove satisfactory. Daylight type glasses with a yellow tint may be suitable for outdoor play. For most other activities and for domed stadiums untinted lenses are undoubtedly satisfactory.

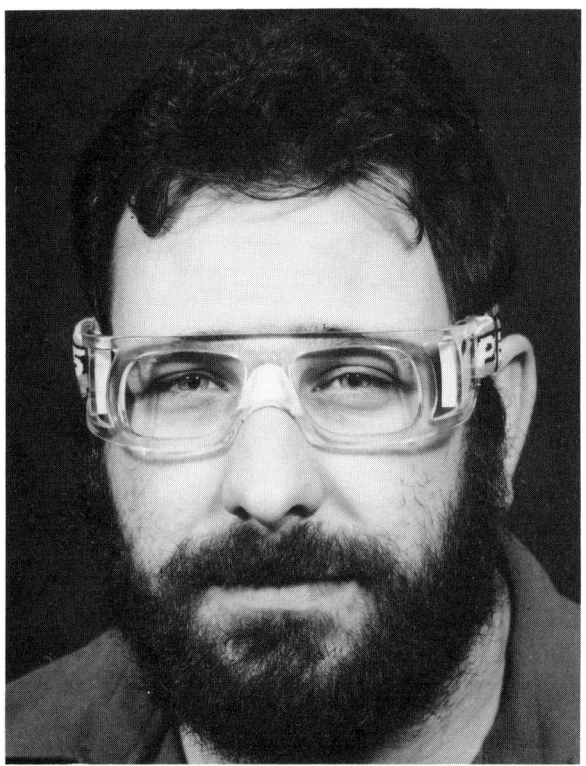

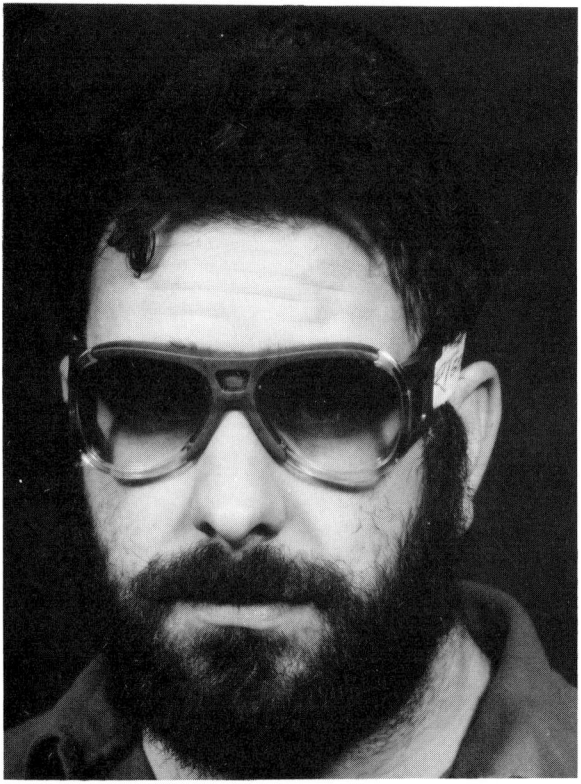

Figure 4-2. Sports spectacles shown are Rec Specs® (top), and Liberty Goggles® (bottom).

In general, professional football players tend to prefer wearing visual correction which provides their best possible corrected visual acuity. Professional football players do not, in general, like playing with uncorrected visual defects. This may be related to the fact that these athletes are individuals who have succeeded in a long and arduous process of selection of the fittest and the best. It would seem that if those who reach the top wish to see better, those who are striving to do their best should do likewise. That is, the developing player would emulate the professional.

The visual acuity level that is required for football is not well-established. The quarterback and ends tend to be the most sensitive about visual difficulties, but all football players with whom I have dealt, seem to prefer to see the very best that they can. For example, to even *see* the football at a distance of eighty yards away requires 20/20 vision.

Ocular motility plays a significant factor with the football player. As with all athletic endeavors and in most endeavors in life, inadequate motility causing diplopia or double vision is extremely disabling. Constant double vision should be a disqualifying ocular factor for playing football at any level. Intermittent double vision could also be a problem, but if diplopia is not elicited under usual playing conditions it should not be a problem for the player. Fatigue can contribute to diplopia, but the adrenalin level associated with active participation in sports tends to negate this factor. The ultimate expression of normal ocular motility and binocular cooperation is stereopsis or depth perception. Stereopsis allows us to see things in depth; that is, the object of regard is seen apart from the surround. Seeing things in depth allows us to react appropriately and accurately with our environment. A simple test of depth and its implications can be demonstrated. Have a person sitting opposite you hold a pencil at its point with the eraser pointing downward. You take a similar pencil holding it by its point with the eraser pointing upward. The two pencils should be vertically aligned with the erasers touching. Now move the pencil abruptly two or three inches to the side and one or two inches downward. After demonstrating the moving pencil, instruct your partner to place his pencil eraser on yours after you have abruptly moved your pencil as described above, with a quick, direct, and accurate movement. When he has accomplished this, continue the motion varying directions from side to side and back and forth five or six times. A person with normal, binocular depth perception will be able to quickly and accurately relocate his pencil eraser to touch yours. The person without depth perception will take two to three times as long to locate and touch your eraser tip and will do so only after making several false movements. Abnormal depth perception or lack of depth perception can be demonstrated by asking your normal partner to now close one eye and then attempt to repeat the test. With a normal individual, there will be a great difference between the binocular, depth perception response and the monocular, lack of depth perception response. Although the individual who has lived chronically with one eye and lacks depth perception can accommodate by using monocular cues, any person lacking depth perception will in no way be able to emulate the performance of one with normal depth perception.

While it is a very important plus factor to have depth perception and stereopsis, it would be inappropriate to discourage an otherwise talented player just because depth perception was lacking. It might be better to see what a person can do with the ability that he has. If the job is too difficult, it won't be long before the player realizes his own limitations. On a personal note, I know of a young medical student who had typical male red-green color deficiency (color blindness). This is a condition which affects 8 percent of males. He was advised by a senior ophthalmologist to select a field of medicine other than ophthalmology for specialty study. The young man had already selected ophthalmology and decided to go ahead against the unsolicited but, nonetheless, forceful advice of the older ophthalmologist. The young medical student completed his residency and continued on to a very successful career in ophthalmology as a surgeon, researcher, and educator.

The presence of retinal disease, particularly in the form of retinal holes, lattice degeneration, and other factors which could lead to retinal detachment should disqualify a participant from strenuous contact sports. While boxing would be the worst, football, diving, wrestling, and several other contact sports should also be included. I have seen several professional athletes with retinal holes in the periphery of the retina which were of a definite predetachment type. These players with highly myopic eyes had had, in some cases, either prophylactic or therapeutic peripheral retinal cryotherapy treatment. If the individual insists on playing, the retina should be watched very closely and the athlete should be adequately warned of the greatly increased risk of traumatic retinal detachment. Amateur or recreational players should be discouraged from engaging in any rough contact sport such as football if retinal holes or breaks which could lead to detachment are present. It is probably not feasible to obtain a detailed peripheral retinal exam as a preplaying screening evaluation on all recreational amateur players. However, a high index of suspicion for such a problem should exist if high myopia, history of visual floaters, or other predisposing factors for retinal detachment are uncovered.

Any individual with amblyopia or decreased vision in one eye from any cause should consider the use of safety glasses as eye protection when engaging in football. Protection is even more important in sports such as basketball, but eye injuries certainly can and do occur in the course of a football game. Eye injuries in football are related to either jolt and concussion, foreign bodies such as fingers, or corneal abrasions due to smaller flying objects.

In a 1984 Colt's regular season game, two players received significant eye injuries on the same play from a similar type of action produced by the same assailant. During a brief altercation brought about because a defensive end thought he was being held by an offensive tackle, the offensive tackle was struck with a long fingernail which was thrust between the globe and the inferior orbital rim. The fingernail in the inferior orbital area caused a tearing type lid laceration. A second player who joined the fray from the sideline was struck by the same defensive end in an identical manner producing an identical injury. Both players were removed immediately to the locker room. Both players complained of extremely blurred vision, one had nausea, and both complained of diplopia or double vision with the second object on top of the real object. One player received x-rays which proved to be negative for blowout fracture. The offensive tackle had persisting diplopia and was held out of the remainder of the game. The second player returned to action in the second half. Both players required butterfly bandage closure of the lid lacerations.

On query after the game, both injured players described their assailant's fingernail as being approximately one inch long. A letter to the supervisor of referees suggesting that players be checked for fingernail length resulted in no action being taken. However, in the interest of eye safety such a rule would be beneficial in my opinion.

The use of a cage type face guard provides good facial and eye protection for most football players. Theoretically, those players who wear a simpler face mask such as those worn by many kickers, quarterbacks, and receivers run an increased risk of facial injury including eye injury (Fig. 4-3).

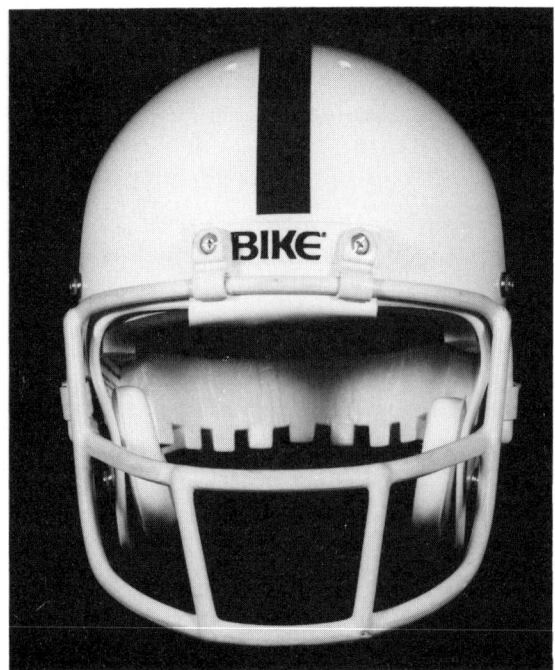
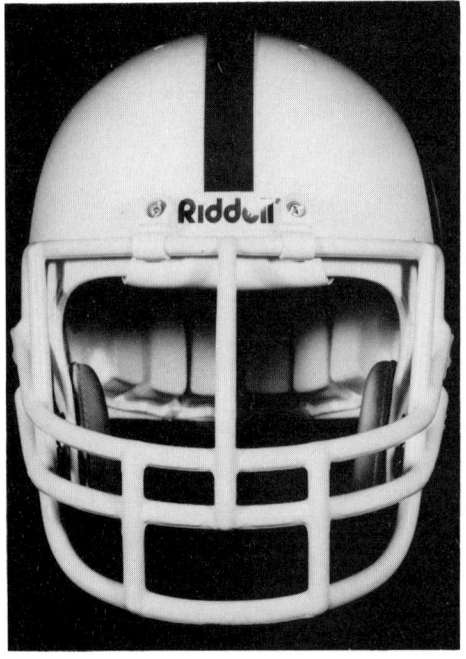
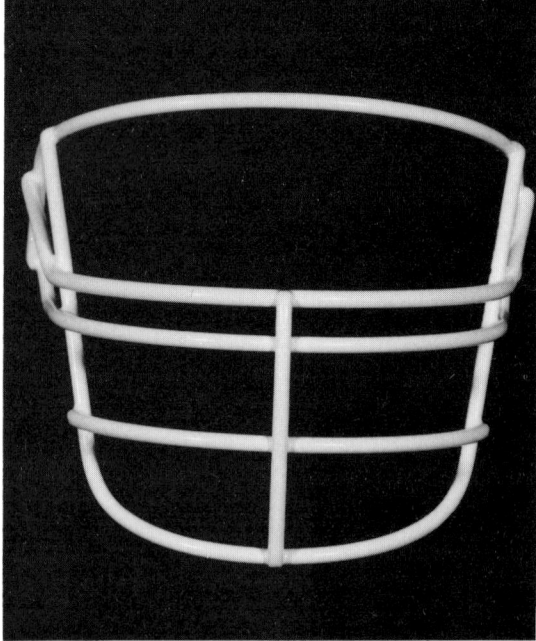

Figure 4-3. Top: Face mask used by quarterbacks, kickers and wide receivers. Clear viewing area provides an unobstructed view.
Bottom left: Cage-type face mask worn by interior linemen. Note heavy bars.
Bottom right: Newer, narrower bars on a cage-type face mask with clear viewing aperature.

The face mask may be augmented in special cases by a clear plastic shield covering the upper half of the inner aspect of the cage. This has been used for players who have been convalescent from corneal abrasions (Fig. 4-4).*

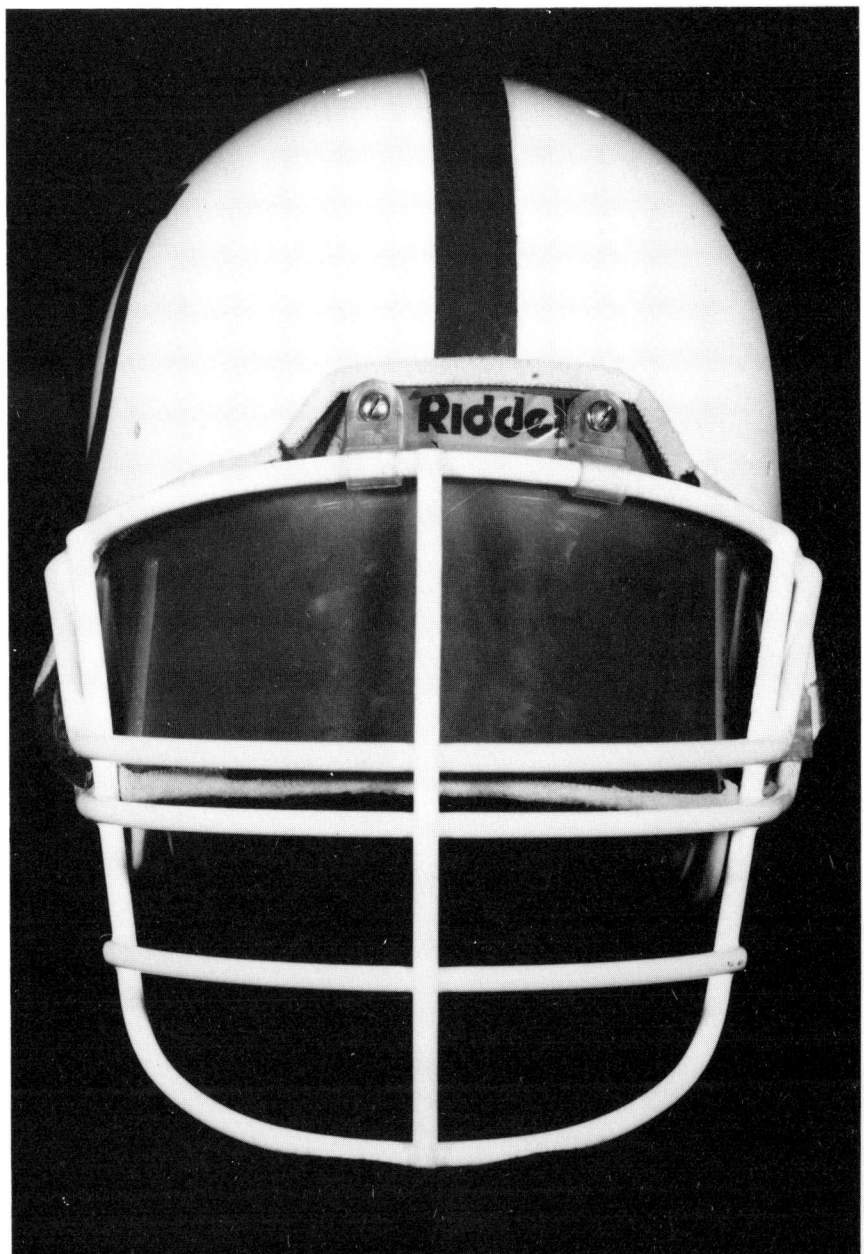

Figure 4-4. Full cage mask with plastic shield to protect the eyes. Worn by a lineman who had a recent corneal abrasion.

---

*This face mask was fabricated by Hunter Smith, head trainer of the Indianapolis Colts Football team.

One unusual problem occurred with regard to the face mask. A tight end noted occasional difficulty with his ocular alignment particular at the distance. On careful testing he was noted to have an intermittent exotropia, divergence excess type. The center bar of his face mask was enough of a dissociating factor to cause the intermittent exotropia at distance to become a manifest exodeviation at times. Newer face cages are constructed of thinner bars.

An unusual injury in football occurred with Fred Arbanas, a tight end for the Kansas City Chiefs in the 1960s. An off season injury caused him to ultimately lose effective vision in one eye. In spite of this, he was able to play effectively for several years with monocular vision. He was an example of a highly motivated person playing over an injury.

Another highly successful Superbowl quarterback was able to attain great success in spite of having a small angle esotropia some amblyopia or poor vision in one eye. He has only peripheral fusion with significantly decreased stereopsis or depth perception. This player was tried with glasses and prisms, but achieved most of his success while using neither.

The trainer's kit for sideline eye care for football players should include the following: Proparacaine Hydrochloride .5 percent for topical anesthesia, dry flourescein strips to stain for corneal abrasions, a penlight with a blue filter cap for inspection of the external eye (the blue filter cap for evaluation for flourescein staining), eye patches, tape, butterfly bandages, cyclopentolate hydrochloride 1 percent for dilating a pupil after a corneal abrasion, sodium sulfacetamide 10 percent drops, and also Neosporin solution for individuals who might be allergic to sulfa, sterile cotton tip applicators, surgical loupes for magnification, and antifogging compound for spectacle lenses. Other useful items are found in the general training kit. These include oral analgesics, and ice for contusion.

It is important to remember that if a player should sustain a "black eye" it could possibly be the harbinger of significant, serious eye pathology. This ranges from subluxation or dislocation of the lens to hyphema (blood in the anterior chamber) to anterior chamber angle recession, to retinal detachment. Any patient with hyphema should be restricted from activity until the hyphema has cleared. Preferably, no contact should be undertaken until at least five days after the injury. Black athletes should be tested for sickle-cell traitor disease in cases of hyphema. The implications of hyphema with sickling trait or disease are much more serious than those without.

The practice of painting the upper cheek with black is based on the notion that this will reduce reflected glare from the cheeks (Fig. 4-5). That this is effective is very doubtful, and I strongly suspect that the practice has more psychological than real benefit. The practice may make the player appear a lot more menacing not unlike the use of "war-paint" by savages. It is especially unlikely that the darkly complexioned black athlete would derive benefit, however, they do use it in some cases. If such a practice were useful it would seem that tennis players would be prime beneficiaries but the fact that they do not employ this practice suggests that the whole concept may be related to the macho image rather than better performance.

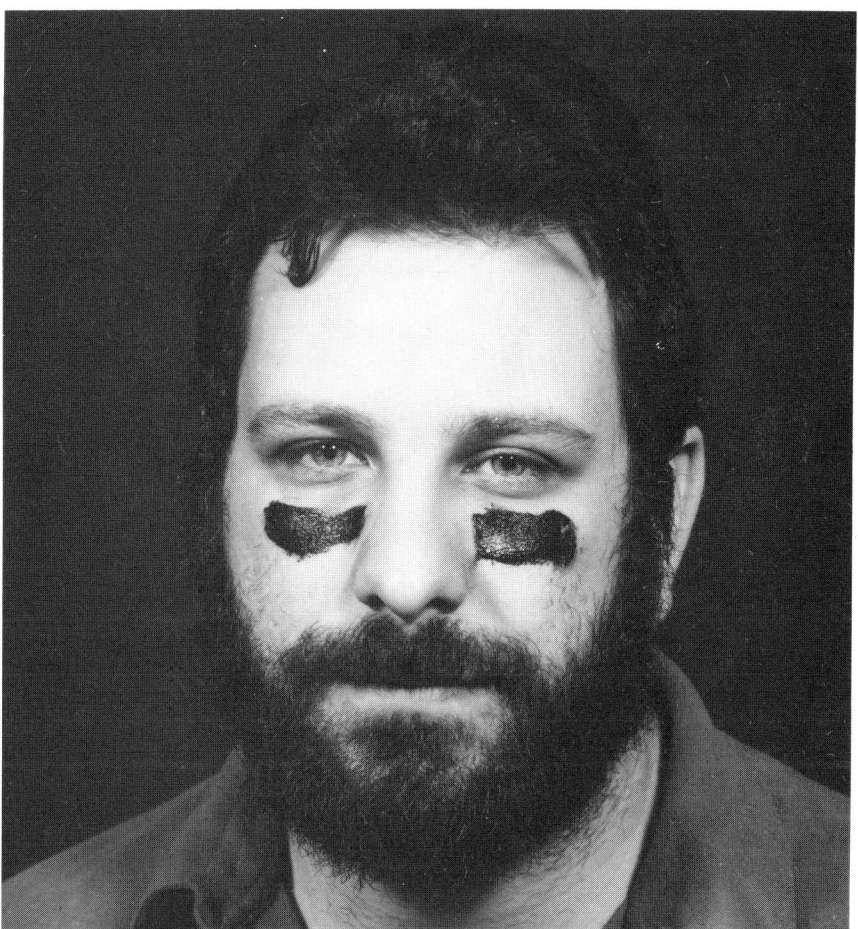

Figure 4-5. Nonglare cream applied to the cheeks as a common practice of questionable value.

In summary, visual needs in football vary with the position. No player should be denied the opportunity to participate on the basis of his visual acuity or other ocular functions, but individuals with retinal disease and impending detachment should be discouraged from football as well as other contact sports. Most football players prefer to play with their best corrected visual acuity. In most cases this is accomplished with the use of soft contact lenses. Soft contact lenses of the oxygen permeable type which are somewhat rigid are the most satisfactory. Stereopsis and depth perception are definitely attributes for the football player, but they are not essential. This is particularly so for players in other than the skill positions. These include the interior linemen and most special teams' players. All individuals who play football should have a thorough baseline ophthalmologic exam. Injuries should be treated appropriately and promptly. Return to play, particularly in instances of hyphema or retinal damage should be subject to complete resolution and should be done under the supervision of an ophthalmologist.

CHAPTER 5

PUGILISM

Louis D. Pizzarello and Barry Jordan

FEW SPORTS provoke the heated outcry like that against boxing. Calls for the elimination of the sport have appeared sporadically in the past.[1,2,3] The medical community, committed to the relief of suffering, finds itself pitted against groups who see the merits of legitimate fisticuffs. The resolution of this situation seems years away. Ophthalmologists are occasionally drawn into the fracas when eye injury and blindness result.

OCULAR INJURY

Boxing exposes the visual system to injury at several levels, including the ocular adnexa, globe, periocular orbital structures, optic nerves and tracts, intracranial nerves, and occipital cortex. Blunt trauma can have a terrifying impact on any or all of these structures. The ophthalmologist needs to be aware of the potential of direct injury as well as that which can occur as long-term sequelae, many years after an active boxing career has ended.

Similar to other sports, boxers are also susceptible to foreign objects lodging in the conjunctival sac or becoming embedded in the cornea. Particulate matter can easily adhere to a boxer's glove, especially after a fall to the canvas, and inadvertently be introduced into the eye of the opponent. Therefore, it is particularly important for the referee to wipe the gloves clean after a boxer has been knocked down. The removal of foreign matter can usually be obtained by gentle irrigation with saline or water or by simply wiping the object away. However, if a foreign body is embedded in the cornea it may require removal using topical anesthesia and the appropriate instruments.

The delicate structures of the eyeball are particularly susceptible to the pummeling blows of the fist. Current gloves, with thumbs, gain easy access to the relatively open lateral approach. Injury may be confined to the cornea with mild abrasion, although folds in Descemet's membrane have been reported after a boxing injury.[1] Conjunctival hemorrhage is sometimes seen after such trauma. Hyphema and angle recession are particularly severe sequelae of pugilism. Palmer et al.[4] examined a group of fifty-five ex-boxers and found angle recessions in 8.2 percent of eyes, a prevalence far higher than that expected in the general population. Interestingly, none of the patients had glaucoma. Importantly, the average follow-up after the final bout in this group was thirty-three years. Wolfe and Zimmerman[5] demonstrated that the glaucoma resulting from angle recession can occur many decades after the initial injury. Frequently the true diagnosis of recession can only be made on gonioscopy soon after the injury. A previous history of boxing should alert the ophthalmologist to look carefully for angle recession. Doggart mentions more severe damage to the ciliary body leading to chronic hypotony and even phthisis bulbi.[1]

Traumatic cataracts may result from blunt ocular trauma and have been reported to occur in boxing. The exact frequency of traumatic cataracts is unknown. Albaugh[6] reported 38 boxers with cataracts. Ten cases were bilateral and 4 cases disappeared spontaneously. Traumatic cataracts may be associated with other ocular lesions such as traumatic iritis, lid ecchymosis, macular contusion, vitreous hemorrhage, and retinal detachment. Although not reported in the Albaugh series, ocular contusion may break zonular attachments to the lens with resultant subluxation or dislocation of the lens.

Retinal detachment in fighters has received a great deal of publicity recently. The case of Sugar Ray Leonard has brought not only retinal detachment to the sports page but also the relative merits of various treatment strategies. Handicapping of various surgeons' successes is soon to follow. In the series of 55 ex-boxers gathered by Palmer, 7 eyes had retinal detachment, quite a significant rate. Albaugh reported a very poor rate of reattachment in the early 1950s,[6] with 1 out of 29 detachments successfully treated. In their series of retinal injury in boxers, Macguire and Benson[7] treated 8 cases of retinal detachment, 4 had macular involvement. Decreased visual acuity was noted in 7 boxers and the eighth boxer noted peripheral visual field loss. Other presenting symptoms included photopsias (light flashes) in 2 and entopsias (floaters) in one. Associated vitreoretinal pathology included posterior vitreous detachments in 5, 3 had a significant hemorrhage, and 2 had an avulsed vitreous base. Fortunately for Sugar Ray, the success rates have improved in the recent past. Choroidal hemorrhage is another frequently encountered entity in all series of fighters. The adage "When you see a pair of cauliflower ears, look out for cauliflower choroid" is an apt one.[1]

ADNEXAL INJURIES

The periorbital structures are favorite targets for boxers. Since the forehead is highly vascularized, there is significant blood loss from these wounds. The supraorbital areas, where the skin is stretched over bone, are sites for frequent laceration. Not only are such wounds psychologically disquieting, but the flow of blood into the eyes frequently obstructs vision to the opponent's advantage. One-third of boxers had scars over the right eye and over half over the left eye in Palmer's series.

The suggested treatment for these periorbital wounds at ringside is application of a swab soaked in 1:1,000 acqueous epinephrine applied directly to the wound and covered with a thin film of Vaseline.® This can be performed by the boxer's trainer at ringside. Later, the fight surgeon can suture the wound appropriately.

Orbital fractures are not uncommon in boxing. These fractures may lead to compromise of the extraocular muscles and result in diplopia. As one boxer, Bill Softly, said, "Yes, I saw two chaps in the ring and I hit the one that isn't there and the one that isn't there hits me."[1] The blow out fracture may be associated with diplopia on upward gaze, restricted movement of the globe, enopthalmos, downward displacement of the globe, and anesthesia or hypesthesia in the distribution of the infraorbital branch of the maxillary nerve. The medial wall fracture may produce a communication between the ethmoid sinus and the orbit that may result in subcutaneous emphysema. Subcutaneous emphysema can be precipitated by blowing the nose. Similar to the blow out fracture, the medial wall fracture can be associated with diplopia if the medial rectus muscle is entrapped or damaged. Ophthalmoparesis, in the absence of orbital fracture or evidence of injury to the central nervous system (CNS), should alert the physician to direct trauma to the extraocular muscles and/or nerves. Bruising of the extraocular muscles can result in temporary diplopia, that responds to a few days of rest.[8]

Fractures around the eye can also compromise the nasolacrimal duct leading to epiphora. Stelland has reported severence of both superior and inferior canaliculi from a punch.[9] Not uncommonly, the elder patient with epiphora will give a history of pugilism in the past.

BRAIN INJURY

Acute and chronic brain injury in boxing may have a direct or indirect effect on the visual system. Acute brain injuries include subdural hematomas, epidural hematomas, brain contusion, intracerebral hemorrhage, and subarachnoid hemorrhage, whereas the punch-drunk syndrome, also known as chronic traumatic encephalopathy, is the prototype for long-term neurological sequelae of boxing. The punch-drunk syndrome may include any combination of dementia or behavioral changes, cerebellar findings, Parkinsonian features, or pyramidal tract dysfunction.[9] Intracranial hemorrhage can directly involve the brainstem nuclei and cause various cranial nerve palsies or intracranial hemorrhage can directly disrupt the optic tracts and radiations or the occipital cortex resulting in visual field defects. The indirect effect of brain injury on the visual system may include subhyloid retinal hemorrhages as seen in subarachnoid hemorrhage or various neurophthalmological abnormalities associated with increased intracranial pressure. These consequences of increased intracranial pressure may include papilledema, optic atrophy, sixth nerve palsies as a false localizing sign, and incomplete or complete third nerve palsies secondary to uncal herniation. Chronic brain injury in boxing may be associated with nystagmus or limitations of upward gaze.[9] Ross et al.[10] reported cerebral atrophy and EEG changes in fighters with severity correlated to the number of bouts fought. The tragedy of the punch-drunk syndrome was brought to the fore by the publicity surrounding the predicament of Mohammed Ali. The outcry against boxing has grown. The editor of the *Journal of the American Medical Association* has called for the banning of the sport.[2] Unfortunately, such pleas have appeared in the past, with seemingly little impact.[1]

PREVENTION OF EYE INJURIES

Periodic ophthalmological examinations represent one of the best methods to prevent eye injuries in boxing. All boxers should undergo an eye examination at least on an annual basis and preferably before each fight. Whether the routine eye examination should be performed by an ophthalmologist has been controversial. The most cost effective approach would be a complete annual eye examination performed by an ophthalmologist and the routine prefight eye examination conducted by the ringside physician. The advantage of the involvement of the ophthalmologist would be primarily to prevent retinal detachment by the early detection of retinal tears. Another advantage would be the prevention of glaucoma by routine measurements of intraocular pressures.

The introduction of the thumbless or thumb-tied glove has been a major safeguard in the prevention of eye injuries. Although far from being universally accepted, the thumbless glove was invented in hope of decreasing thumbing injuries to the eye. Gloves with thumbs gain easy access into the orbit which can result in some of the ocular injuries mentioned above. Another advantage of the thumbless glove is the prevention of hyperextension injuries to the thumb.

The ringside physician is also of vital importance in the prevention of eye injuries in boxing. Knowledge of when to terminate a fight when a boxer is at risk of serious eye injury is crucial. There are certain medical situations that result in the termination of a bout. If a boxer sustains a "through and through" laceration of the eyelid, the fight should be stopped. Boxing competitions where a boxer sustains a periorbital hematoma which completely closes the eye should also be discontinued. The rationale for this is twofold. First, if a boxer experiences occluded vision on the side of the injury, he may not visualize punches coming from the blind side. Second, if a boxer can't see out, then the physician cannot see in the eye and properly examine it for any ocular pathology.

Protective headgear is also instrumental in the prevention of eye injuries in boxing. Although headgear does not decrease the frequency of knockouts (knockouts are usually the result of acceleration-deceleration injuries), it can reduce trauma to the periorbital structures from direct blows and from head butts.

Injury has also been reported from outside the ring. Verdenthal[11] has presented a tragic case of bilateral retinal detachment in an infant who has been the object of child abuse. Ocular injuries following fisticuffs or beatings are seen by nearly every ophthalmologist. As long as man continues to physically abuse his fellow, traumatic eye disease will be found.

REFERENCES

1. Doggart, James H: The impact of boxing upon the visual apparatus. *Arch. Ophth, 54:* 161-169, 1955.
2. Lundberg, G.D.: Boxing should be banned in civilized countries. *JAMA, 249:* 250, 1983.
3. Von Allen, Maurice: The deadly degrading sport. *JAMA, 249:* 250, 1983.
4. Palmer, Edward; Lieberman, Theodore and Burns, Stanley: Contusion angle deformities in prizefighters. *Arch. Ophth, 94:* 225, 1976.
5. Wolfe, S.M., and Zimmerman, L.E.: Chronic secondary glaucoma associated with retroplacement of iris root and deepening of the anterior angle secondary to contusion. *Am. J. Ophthalm, 54:* 547, 1962.
6. Albaugh, C.H.: Eye problems in boxing. *J. Internat. Coll. Surg, 17:* 191-194, 1952.
7. Macguire, J.I. and Benson, W.E.: Retinal injury and detachment in boxers. *JAMA, 255:* 2451-2453, 1986.
8. Whiteson, A.L., Injuries in professional boxing; their treatment and prevention. *Practitioner, 225:* 1056-1057, 1981.
9. Ross, Ronald, J., Cole, M., Thompson, J., and Kim, Kyung: Boxers-Computed tomography, EEG and neurological evaluation. *JAMA, 249:* 211-213, 1983.
10. Roberts, A.H.: *Brain damage in boxers.* London, Pitman Scientific Publishing Co., 1969.
11. Weidenthal, Daniel T., and Levin, Daniel B: Retinal detachment in a battered infant. *Am. J. Ophthalm, 81:* 725-727, 1976.

CHAPTER 6

AQUATIC SPORTS

DAVID H. ABRAMSON AND RICHARD A. MCDONOUGH

MANY SPORTS take place in an aquatice environment. Competitive swimming, diving, water ballet, and water polo all occur in swimming pools. Scuba diving, snorkeling, and recreational swimming frequently take place outdoors in fresh or salt water. The human eye has to adjust to the watery world in two ways. First, the new ambient surroundings are different and second, visual function and needs are dramatically altered. At times the sportsman needs good vision and at other times vision is much less a problem. This chapter deals with particular problems associated with eyes and water sports.

While one swims, the eyes are exposed to and interact with a variety of substances (both organic and inorganic) which are present in pool water. Undoubtedly, the first of these substances to come to mind when associating pool water and the eyes is the disinfectant, chlorine. The most widely used and best known chemical for the treatment of pool water, chlorine is labeled the source of eye irritation in swimmers. As we shall see later, it is not necessarily chlorine which causes the eye irritation, but other related and unrelated factors. To better understand chlorine's effect on the eyes, one must first understand its role in the swimming pool environment.

The halogen, although one of the most widely distributed elements, is not found in a free state in nature. Instead, it exists predominantly in combination with sodium, potassium, calcium, and magnesium. Elemental chlorine is a heavy gas of greenish-yellow coloration which functions as an oxidizer in most of its chemical reactions. The reason for chlorine's powerful oxidizing ability is an outer shell of seven electrons in its atomic structure.

When calcium is treated with gaseous chlorine and sodium chloride is electrolyzed, calcium hypochlorite and sodium hypochlorite are formed in the respective reactions. These solids, as well as gaseous chlorines are the most common forms in which chlorine is administered to a swimming pool. This provides a basis through which we can examine the chemical reactions involved in chlorination.

When chlorine is administered to a body of water, a certain amount of the chlorine will be consumed by water impurities. This is known as the water's chlorine demand. Because of the chlorine's strong oxidizing ability (derived from its electron configuration), it readily reacts with inorganic reducing substances such as ferrous iron ($Fe.^{++}$), manganous manganese ($Mn.^{++}$), nitrates ($NO_{2\text{-}}$),[1] and hydrogen sulfide (H_2S), as well as organic material (other than amines). The result of these reactions is the chlorine atoms' reduction to chloride and, thereby losing their oxidizing and disinfecting properties.

The chlorine that remains after the water's chlorine demand has been fulfilled, is known as residual available chlorine. It is this chlorine that will react with any further inorganic or organic material entering the pool environment. Residual available chlorine exists essentially as free available chlorine or combined available chlorine. Since elemental chlorine (Cl_2) is present for only a moment within the normal pH zone, the term "free available chlorine" refers most often to hypochlorous acid (HOCl) and the hypochlorite ion (OCl-) in practice. Provided chlorine demand is satisfied and there is no ammonia or nitrogenous compounds present, free available chlorine exists in water; the distribution of the three forms depending on pH. When ammonia and/or other nitrogenous compounds are introduced into pool water, chlorine combines with them to form chloramines or N-chloro compounds. This is known as "combined available chlorines."

DISINFECTION

Although many factors are involved with chlorine disinfection, pH is by far the most important one in determining chlorine efficiency. At pH values below 2 (of which very little study has been done), a small percentage of the chlorine appears to be in elemental form and is quite effective. Between pH 2 and 6, a major portion of the chlorine is in the form of hypochlorous acid. Increase in pH from 5 to 10 produces a two-hundred fold decrease in germicidal action due to the increasing presence of hypochlorite ion. Hypochlorite acid is the primary disinfectant.

Hypochlorite ions are far less effective, therefore the power of free chlorine residual decreases with increasing pH.

Bactericidal action of combined available residual chlorine is significantly less than that of free available residual chlorine. Although chloramines have been known to provide the prolonged stability of chlorine, to effect rapid bactericidal action a contact time of 100 times longer and a concentration 25 times greater than that of free available residual chlorine is required.

Purposeful disinfection of water has the specific mission of killing those organisms which may spread infection in an aquatic environment. Prevention of direct transmission of disease (ocular infections in particular) to man through water is of paramount importance. Organisms in water must be destroyed. Also, there is an increased risk of respiratory or skin diseases to persons swimming in pools.

While there are various theories as to chlorine's bacteriocidal mode of action, the enzyme trace substance theory is generally accepted today. Chlorine, as an exceptionally active inhibitor of sulfhydryl enzymes, reacts with sulfhydryl groups and causes cell death by interruption of essential metabolic systems. This may occur at several loci, causing termination of glucose oxidation and loss of cell viability. Chlorine in the minimal concentration required for complete inhibition of glucose oxidation is sufficient to sterilize a bacterial suspension. Triose phosphate dehydrogenase (an oxidation enzyme) is particularly chlorine sensitive.

When exposed to chlorine concentrations necessary for enzyme inhibition, bacterial spores lose their ability to oxidize glucose, but are not killed. The amounts of chlorine required to inhibit glucose oxidation in spores and negative cells is the same. Spores are able to survive where vegetative cells die because of their ability to produce more of the susceptible enzyme. In vegetative cells, the gene controlling the enzyme's synthesis is more accessible than in the spore, and it is thereby inactivated.

A brief sidetrack to mention iodine and bromine will complete our knowledge of swimming pool disinfection. Iodine is added to water in the form of potassium iodide which, when combined with a minimal amount of chlorine, releases free iodine. Even with a small applied dosage, iodine treated pools are equal in quality to those treated with chlorine. No odors, taste, or eye irritations have been attributed to exposure to iodine-treated pool water. Because of the risk to iodine sensitive individuals, iodine has not gained wide acceptance as a swimming pool disinfectant. Bromochlordimethydantoin, a synthetic compound, has been used as a bromine source. When it comes in contact with water, bromine and chlorine are liberated from the compound. The free bromine level is maintained for much longer periods of time than the free chlorine level which diminishes rapidly. When bromamines are found, bromine activity is maintained. The maintenance of a residual level of 2 ppm. of bromine effects virtual elimination of coliforns, enterococci, streptococcus viridans, and staphylococci. No viruses have been isolated from bromine treated water. Even very high concentrations of bromine (9ppm.) do not produce an odor or irritate mucous membranes.

Effects on the Eye

There are many sources for ocular irritation from swimming pools. These include chemical irritation, mechanical irritation from floating substances and filters, corneal edema, superficial punctate keratitis, and ocular infections. Corneal abrasions, especially in water polo players, are common.

The most common and prevalent finding is corneal edema in swimmers who have been in fresh water swimming pools. After thirty-four minutes of swimming without goggles, 68 percent of one series of individuals demonstrated corneal edema.[5] (At chlorine concentrations of 1.0 to 1.5 PPM and pH 7.5). Although slit lamp examination revealed that 94 percent of these volunteers had corneal epithelial erosions in a punctate or linear pattern, no subject showed a measurable decrease in visual acuity. The symptoms were halos and rainbows and usually resolved within thirty minutes. Corneal edema does not change significantly when either pH or clorine concentrations are changed. The corneal edema which is so prevalent in fresh water pools is also seen in nonchlorinated fresh water, but rarely in salt water (which is isotonic).

Chlorine will cause some ocular discomfort. Although increasing concentrations of chlorine do cause a slight increase in eye irritation, the discomfort is more related to pH than chlorine concentration. A pH of 7.0 produces a notable increase in eye irritation when compared to a pH of 8.0 at the same concentrations of chlorine. Rises in pH have also been found in fresh water lakes, secondary to acid rain.[6]

Another important cause of ocular irritation is the chlorine derived chloramines. These are mostly formed from the chlorine combinations with ammonia compounds found on the skin and from urine. The chloramines collect as insoluble gases on the surface of the pool, and are very irritating to the corneal epithelium.

Mechanical factors, such as currents from the filtered water and fine floating debris also contribute to corneal irritation. It has been suggested that the friction of water against the cornea with disruption of the tear film may also contribute to corneal erosions and edema.

Corneal abrasions in water polo players are not usual, and are not accidental. Many players have been taught to aim for the cornea and cause an abrasion in the hope of causing a player to withdraw from competition. Although anesthetics are not allowed in amateur competitions, many coaches do carry topical anesthetics and even fluorescein strips to examine and treat their players at poolside.

Infections

The toxic effect of chlorine on a variety of organisms has been studied and is presented in Table 6-1. It is obvious that chlorine is very toxic to a variety of algae, fungi, nematodes, protozoa, plants, bacteria, bacteriophage, and viruses. To some extent, these noxious effects are dependent upon temperature, pH and chlorine concentration. For example, at a pH of 7.0 *Clostridium botulinum* is destroyed after only thirty seconds exposure to 0.5 PPM at 25°C (comparable to a swimming pool). *Streptococcus fecalis* is destroyed at the same temperature, same levels of chlorine at pH of 7.5. *Mycobacterium tuberculosis,* on the other hand, required 50 PPM at 50-60°C to be destroyed.

Plants, frogs, and even fish are killed after relatively short periods of exposure to chlorinated water. It would appear that if a patient with active conjunctivitis entered a swimming pool, the chlorinated water would probably be beneficial to the infection and even help in preventing the further exposure and transmission of the infection to others.

Epidemics of conjunctivitis in swimmers are, however, well-recognized and well-supported. These epidemics have repeatedly been attributed to Adenoviruses of different types, despite the fact that Adenovirus is inactive after three minutes exposure to chlorinated water.[7] The reason Adenoviruses have caused these infections is that faulty equipment, inadequate chlorination, or human error in maintaining swimming pools has been shown to have occurred, leading to epidemics of infection. It is of interest that many different Adenovirus types have been associated with swimming pool conjunctivitis. Recounting their epidemics is instructive.

Table 6-1
BIOCIDAL EFFECT OF FREE AVAILABLE CHLORINE ON VARIOUS ORGANISMS

Organism	pH	Temp. (°C)	Exposure Time	ppm Av. Cl_2	Biocidal Results
ALGAE					
Chlorella varegata	7.8	22	—	2.0	Growth Controlled
Gomphonema parvulum	8.2	22	—	2.0	Growth Controlled
Microcystis aeruginosa	8.2	22	—	2.0	Growth Controlled
BACTERIA					
Achromobacter metalcaligenes	6.0	21	15 seconds	5.0	100%
Bacillus anthracis	7.2	22	120 minutes	2.3-2.4	100%
B. globigii	7.2	22	120 minutes	2.5-2.6	99.99%
Clostridium botulinum toxin type A	7.0	25	30 seconds	0.5	100%
Escherichia coli	7.0	20-25	1 minute	0.055	100%
E. typhosa	8.5	20-25	1 minute	0.1-0.29	100%
Mycobacterium tuberculosis	8.4	50-60	30 seconds	50	100%
Pseudomonas fluoresceins IM	6.0	21	15 seconds	5.0	100%
Shigella dysenteriae	7.0	20-25	3 minutes	0.046-0.055	100%
Staphylococcus aureus	7.2	25	30 seconds	0.8	100%
Streptococcus faecalis	7.5	20-25	2 minutes	0.5	100%
All vegetative bacteria	9.0	25	30 seconds	0.2	100%
BACTERIOPHAGE					
S. cremoris phage strain 144F	6.9-8.2	25	15 seconds	25	100%
FISH					
Carassius auratus	7.9	Room	96 hours	1.0	Killed
Daphnia magna	7.9	Room	72 hours	0.5	Killed
FROGS					
Rana pipiens	8.3	21	4 days	10	100%
FUNGI					
Aspergillus niger	10-11	20	30-60 minutes	100	100%
Rhodotorula flava	10-11	20		100	100%

Table 6-1 (continued)

Organism	pH	Temp. (°C)	Exposure Time	ppm Av. Cl$_2$	Biocidal Results
NEMATODES					
C. quadrilabiatus	6.6-7.2	25	30 minutes	95-100	93%
D. nudicapitatus	6.6-7.2	25	30 minutes	95-100	97%
PLANTS					
Cabomba caroliniana	6.3-7.7	Room	4 days	5	100%
Elodea canadensis	6.3-7.7	Room	4 days	5	100%
PROTOZOA					
Endamoeba histolytica cysts	7.0	25	150 minutes	0.08-0.12	99-100%
VIRUSES					
Purified adenovirus 3	8.8-9.0	25	40-50 seconds	0.2	99.8%
Purified Coxsackie A$_2$	6.9-7.1	27-29	3 minutes	0.92-1.0	99.6%
Purified Coxsackie B$_1$	7.0	25	2 minutes	0.31-0.40	99.9%
Purified Coxsackie B$_5$	7.0	25-28	1 minute	0.21-0.30	99.9%
Infectious hepatitis	6.7-6.8	Room	30 minutes	3.25	Protected all 12 volunteers
Purified poliovirus (Mahoney)	7.0	25-28	3 minutes	0.21-0.30	99.9%
Purified poliovirus (Lensen)	7.4-7.9	19-25	10 minutes	1.0-0.5	Protected all 164 inoculated mice
Purified poliovirus III (Sankett)	7.0	25-28	2 minutes	0.11-0.2	99.9%
Purified Theiler's	6.5-7.0	25-27	5 minutes	4-6	99%

In 1973, an epidemic of acute conjunctivitis occurred in Shawnee Mission, Kansas.[8] Investigation by the CDC revealed that the local junior high school swimming pool was the source of the infection. The filter sump pump filtered the water every eight hours, and automatically chlorinated the water by adding hypochlorite each hour. When the system broke down, the coach noted that the chlorine level was low and manually added chlorine daily. Of swim team members who were exposed to the lower levels of chlorine almost 20 percent came down with illness, while none of the members of the gym class (who swam when chlorine levels were again normal) came down with illness. The safe area for chlorination appeared to be between 0.3 and 1.0 PPM and the unsafe level between 0.0 and 0.3 PPM. Of those who became ill, the most common manifestation was red or pink eyes (100 percent), followed by swollen eyes (75 percent), painful eyes (71 percent), tearing (66 percent), exudate (52 percent), fever (52 percent), headache (46 percent), photophobia (36 percent), crusts (36 percent), lymphadenopathy (34 percent), cough (30 percent), nausea (23 percent), vomiting (11 percent), painful joints (9 percent), sore throat (9 percent), stomachache (5 percent), dizziness (5 percent), diarrhea (5 percent), and earache (5 percent). Adeno-7 was isolated as the cause of the epidemic. The authors pointed out that adenoviruses may come from the eye, pharynx, or anus to cause such epidemics. They reiterated that Adenovirus-3 is known to be inactivated in three minutes, but that the pool in this case was underchlorinated.

Another epidemic was reported from Georgia where Adenovirus-3 was found to be the etiologic agent in a swimming pool-caused epidemic.[9] In this case, the epidemic was traced to a temporary defect in the chlorination system. In these cases, the most common symptoms were sore throat (80 percent), fever (78 percent), anorexia (67 percent), headache (65 percent), nausea (39 percent), chills (37 percent), coughs (37 percent), earache (37 percent), conjunctivitis (35 percent), runny/stuffy nose (35 percent), vomiting (33 percent), myalgia (30 percent), swollen glands (26 percent), sputum (17 percent), diarrhea (11 percent), arthralgia (6 percent), and rash (4 percent). There were no permanent effects in either case. Children under the age of nine appeared to be more susceptible than those ages ten through nineteen who appeared more susceptible than those over the age of twenty.

It has been emphasized that Adenovirus disappears from the conjunctiva after fourteen days, but fecal excretion can continue for thirty days after infection. Isolating the source of the epidemic may be possible at times.

Finally, it must be remembered that epidemics of viral and bacterial conjunctivitis may occur in swimmers through the usual airborne or direct transmission by hands, goggles, and towels.

Swimming goggles and masks come close to the panacea for all ocular problems for swimmers. They prevent exposure of the eye to infectious agents and prevent mechanical disruption of the cornea from water, particles, and fingers. They have been associated with a chemical keratitis.[10] Pressure from the goggles has been associated with supraorbital neuralgia[11] and migraine headaches[12] have also been attributed to swimming goggles. Also several ocular injuries have been reported from goggles that have slipped out of young hands.[13]

Other aquatic sports have peculiar ocular problems. Scuba diving has been associated with problems for hard contact lens wearers.[14] Cotter, however, with extensive testing found no real problem with soft contact lens wear beneath a scuba wash, except lens loss. Diving has been associated with trauma to the eye including a rare case of optic nerve hematoma.[15]

Banned Drops

A recent survey of swimmers revealed that the majority of them use some eye drops after swimming to relieve the irritation caused by swimming pools. Unfortunately, they are using drops which contain ingredients which would automatically disqualify them from Olympic competition. Olympic rules do not distinguish topically used from systemically administered drugs. Thus, drops containing any concentration of topical sympathomimetics may not be used or carried. A partial list of banned drops include:

Vasocon-A
Naphcon-A
Prefin
Prefin-A
Zincfrin
Collyrium with Ephedrine

REFERENCES

1. Block, Seymor S.: *Disinfection, Sterilization and Preservation* (3rd ed.), Phila, Lea & Febiger, 1983.
2. Clark, John William; Viessman Jr., Warren and Hammer, Mark J.: *Water Supply and Pollution Control* (2nd ed.), Scranton, International Textbook Co., 1971.
3. Fair, Gordon M., and Okun, Daniel A.: *Water and Wastewater Engineering: Water Purification and Wastewater Treatment and Disposal,* (vol. 2), New York, Bks Demand UMI, 1968.
4. Hedgecock, L.W.: *Anti-Microbial Agents.* Phila, Lea & Febiger, 1967.
5. Haag, J.R. & Gieser, R.G.: Effects of swimming pool water on the cornea, *JAMA, 249:* 2507, 1983.
6. Basu, P.K.: Acid rain and the eye, *Con Med Assoc J. 125:* 338, 1981.
7. Clarke, N.A. et al: The inactivation of purified type 3 adenovirus in water by chlorine, *Aj J., H&G 64:* 314, 1976.
8. Caldwell, G.G., et al: Epidemic of adenovirus type 7 acute conjunctivitis in swimmers, *Am J Epidemiol, 99:* 230, 1974.
9. Martone, W.J. et al: An outbreak of adenovirus type 3 disease at a private recreation center swimming pool. *Am J Epidemiol, III, 229,* 1980.
10. Wright, W.L.: Scuba diver's delayed toxic epithelial keratopathy form commercial mask defogging agents. *Am J Ophthalmol, 93:* 470, 1982.
11. Jacobson, R.I.: More "goggle headaches": supraorbitol neurolgia. *N Engl J Med, 308:* 1363, 1983.
12. Petstonic, A: Ibid p. 226.
13. F. Jonasson: Swimming goggles causing severe eye injuries. *S Brit Med J, 1:* 881, 1977.
14. Cotter, J.: Soft contact lens testing on fresh water scuba divers. *Contact Lens Med J, 7:* 323, 1981.
15. Jonasson, F. & Cullen, J.: Axonal transport injury caused by diving. *Am J Ophthalmol 94:* 813, 1982.

CHAPTER 7

VISUAL APPROACH TO WINNING TENNIS

HAROLD STEIN, BERNARD SLATT, AND RAYMOND STEIN

CORRECT USE of vision and visual clues are vitally important to playing good tennis. Understanding the visual demands of tennis and identifying the limits of the visual apparatus can contribute to an improved game. In this chapter, we will discuss how to gain maximum benefit from visual clues in order to play winning tennis.

As both ophthalmologists and tennis players, we feel eminently qualified to write this chapter. As tennis players, we range from A to C level in proficiency—Ray Stein has taught at the John Newcombe Tennis Camps and has organized his own instructional tours. Professionally, we share an equal interest in discovering and understanding the physiologic visual mechanisms required to play tennis properly.[1]

It has been relatively easy to dismantle old concepts on the capacity of the eye to track a tennis ball. We believe that understanding the visual elements of tennis is as important as learning the correct grip and racket swing. It is time that ophthalmology was formally involved with tennis in order to bring a little science to the locker room. The familiar slogan, "keep your eye on the ball," imparts misleading and false information. A player who tries to follow the ball all the way to his racket strings cannot make a great return, because the ball is too fast for his eyes to track at such close range. He cannot and should not attempt to see the point of contact between the ball and racket.

In preparing this work, we have drawn from evidence in ocular nystagmography and electromyography of ocular muscles. The basic research is not new, but its application to the game of tennis is fresh.

HOW QUICK IS THE EYE?

The standard ophthalmologic examination is for static vision—both the eyes and the chart are stationary. In tennis, however, everything is moving. To construct the same test model, the subject would have to be running a treadmill, with his eyes constantly moving, trying to locate a fast moving projectile in space, in which the contrast and background are variable.

Thus there is no relationship between seeing well in the traditional sense and having good athletic vision or dynamic visual acuity.[2] It is possible to have excellent stationary visual acuity and poor dynamic visual acuity. Fairground games in which moving ducks have to be "shot" are handled well by few people. Those who are successful have good dynamic visual acuity—the ability to follow a moving target. Such vision requires judgment, experience, contrast, good stationary vision and proper illumination. Few people develop excellent dynamic visual skills because these skills are not demanded every day. With reading, writing, or woodworking, the head and eyes are usually still, as is the object of regard—the papers or the work bench.

Motion can disturb vision.[3,4] Anyone who has tried to read on the subway or the bus knows that motion makes reading difficult. In tennis, returning serve is especially difficult because the player must react to the motion of both the ball and the server.

How well do we see while in motion?[5,6] No one can answer the question. There are no commercial tests to judge the visual thresholds of the eye. Eyecare specialists are far behind cardiologists, who employ a variety of moving stress tests to determine the function of the heart. Aerobics has become part of the medical and general jargon. Everyone understands the need to exercise the heart and lungs, but the tennis athlete who routinely does his body exercises may have inferior dynamic visual acuity. He may constantly see the ball late and make errors in judgment because he cannot cope with the sensory demands of the game.

In actuality, our visual equipment is severely limited to cope with the tough demands of tennis. The eyes follow moving objects very slowly. Move a finger back and forth before your eyes, like a pendulum, keeping in view the half moon at the base of the nail. Speed up the motion. It doesn't take much speed to blur the image of the half moon. Turn the automobile windshield wipers to "fast" and see if your eyes can follow them. They will attempt to follow the motion thrusts and then give up.

Or move a pencil back and forth about 18 inches from a friend's eyes and see how soon his visual tracking movements break down. How effectively would the eyes follow the ball from a fast flat serve?

In tennis, our eyes cannot track a ball unless it is moving extremely slowly. The eye might be able to follow a lob as it arches up and slowly descends, but on the toss for the serve, the velocity of the ball is too great for the eye to follow its ascent. The server looks up first and then tosses the ball into his field of vision. During fast play, the eye cannot follow the ball, because there is no mechanism that allows it to make fast movements and keep the ball in sharp focus.

The eye, however, is capable of fast movements. They are called ocular saccades. We use ocular saccades when we watch a parade, read, or try to track the flight of a high-velocity missile (e.g., a tennis ball). But unfortunately, ocular saccades actually suppress vision, even to the level of legal blindness. When we read, for instance, we shift our eyes quickly from place to place taking in information only when the eyes come to rest. To test this phenomenon, hold up your two fingers twenty inches apart, glance quickly from finger to finger, back and forth; repeat the action in front of a mirror. You will see each index finger as your eyes come to rest, but you will not see your own face in the mirror. An object is in focus only when your eyes are still. Consequently, fast eye movements (ocular saccades) provide information between two points on the trajectory of a tennis ball, but because of visual suppression, they cannot give a player information all the way to the racket.

Tennis is especially difficult because of last-minute, motion demands made on the eyes. If a player has to make a visual correction at the last second for an unanticipated slice ball or crooked bounce, in all probability his return stroke will be poor.

How does the eye track a fast ball? Consider the return of serve. The server's motion reveals which type of serve to expect—flat, slice, or twist. Once the ball is struck, although it cannot be seen clearly, its flight pattern can be estimated with relative ease, provided the receiver does not move as the ball is served. Somewhere near the bounce, the player will lose sight of the ball, as it enters the "zone of fog." The exact point when the ball is lost depends on several important variables: illumination (visibility is more difficult by nightlights than by daylight); color contrasts between the ball and the court (fresh balls should be used for contrast as much as for bounce); the dynamic visual acuity of the player (the occasional or slow tennis player is more easily blinded by speed);

and fitness (fatigue causes a player to see the ball late). As the ball approaches the edge of the player's field of vision, he moves his eyes to focus on the ball and project its probable flight pattern. If the ball hits a pebble, is carried by the wind, or slices in an erratic direction, the chances are the player will make a bad return. His sensory and motor apparatus are not fast enough to make a lightening-quick change to a new position.

Consider the best conditions for making a successful return. The ball is coming directly to the player from a hard, flat serve at a speed he cannot follow. He might make one or two ocular saccades to pick up visual information from a fleeting glimpse of the ball, before abandoning the ball altogether. If he is moving, he will not even attempt fast corrective eye movements. His eyes will remain glued to the point where the ball was last seen clearly. The ability to scan a ball in space takes practice, as in speed-reading. The eyes must be able to take in a great deal of information (visual clues) when, for a millisecond, they freeze fast motion. Frequent and long visual stops are useless in a fast game.

Many mistakes in a game are falsely attributed to a player's lack of concentration and visual discipline. The average tennis player tries unsuccessfully to follow the ball right to the racket strings. He has been admonished from the first lesson, "keep your eye on the ball"—an adage that is repeated over and over again as his skills progress.

The ability of the eye to focus clearly on a high-speed missile depends on the viewer's field of vision. At a great distance (e.g., the broad sweep of the sky) the visual field is enormous. Hence, it is possible to track the flight of a jet airplane moving at the speed of sound with only the slightest eye movement. Or a high-speed chase may be witnessed on a movie screen. Our field of vision is expanded by distance, so that moving objects can be seen clearly regardless of their speed.

Conversely, as an object moves closer, the field of vision gets smaller. If the object is speeding, it requires constant visual adjustment to keep the object in sight. It is a race which the eye is destined to lose. In a narrow visual field, the eye can track an object clearly only when the object is moving slowly.

All athletes playing sports that require hand/eye coordination suffer the same visual handicaps. A baseball batter can easily see the ball thrown from third base to second base, but when the pitcher throws the ball directly at him this visual guidance mechanism fails him. If a professional baseball player could see the ball all the way into the bat, the best ones would bat 1.000 and not .333. Baseball, from the standpoint of the

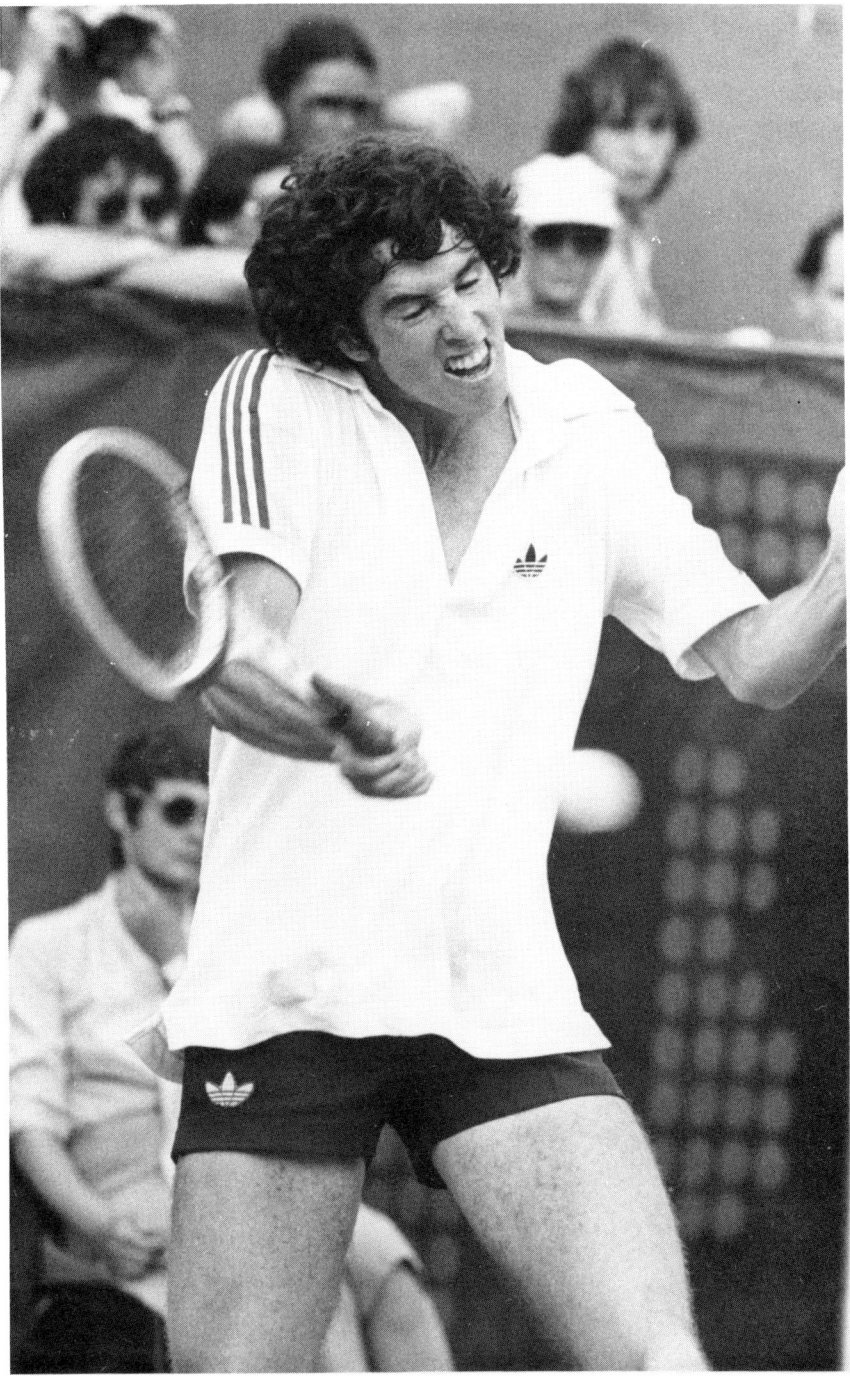

Figure 7-1. Elliot Telcher: Hitting with his eyes closed.

batter, is a consistently high-speed game — all balls travel approximately 70 to 100 miles per hour.

The speed of a tennis ball is not consistent. It varies anywhere from 10 to 80 miles per hour. The velocity is determined by several factors: the skill of the player; the type of shot — serve, volley, and overhead smash are the fastest; position of the receiver — the closer to the net, the faster the ball; and court surface — clay is slowest and grass is fastest. The visual technique for tracking slow and fast balls are quite different. Most players do not make the necessary adjustment to their strokes as predicated by the speed of the ball.

THE ZONE OF FOG

We refer to the area around the point of impact as the blur zone or zone of fog. As the racket swings through the air, only its broad outline can be visualized, but not the gut or other markings. Thus, the blur zone encompasses an area in depth and width the size of the circumference of a half circle inscribed by the backswing, impact, and follow-through, on the player's forehand and backhand sides. For all intents and purposes, hitting the ball is a totally blind act. No one ever sees the ball hit the racket (not even a slow ball), because of the blurring movement of the racket. Unless a player's game is recorded by video tape or high-speed photography, he will never be able to prove conclusively where he hit the ball in relation to his racket or in relation to his body position.

The degree of fog surrounding impact is determined by the dynamic visual acuity of the player, the speed of the ball, and the amount of player motion. The zone becomes denser as the speed of the ball increases and wider if the player is moving. The dynamic visual acuity is variable; it depends on such factors as fitness, freedom from fatigue, judgment, and the player's athletic ability.

We examined 3,000 random action photographs of the professionals, which showed there is a profound disparity between players' ocular hold on a moving ball. Bjorn Borg seemed to have excellent dynamic visual acuity and could track the ball close to the racket. Such players as Jimmy Connors and Vitas Gerulaitus, however, rarely seemed to have their eyes on the ball. Their zone of fog was large, and they compensated for it by looking ahead in the direction the ball was coming from. Obviously a lack of dynamic visual acuity is not a stumbling block to playing great tennis. Most of the professionals we studied seemed to abandon the ball with their eyes as it approached the fog zone.

It is possible to deliberately reduce (but not eliminate) the size of the fog zone by slowing down the game. Most players do this. In the first serve, the receiver may step back to take the ball at a slower velocity which also gives him a longer visual hold on the ball. There is a fundamental risk in adopting this strategy. The farther back a player stations himself, the greater is his displacement from a well-placed ball to a corner of the court. For visual security, he gives up command of the court and is forced to run excessively. By running, he enlarges the zone of fog and thereby defeats the purpose of staying back—visual stability. It is a "Catch 22" of tennis.

Tennis athletes understand little of the function and limitations of the eyes. Even the best players are unaware of the visual judgments they make. In the absence of training programs to help players improve visual acuity, false information is perpetuated by coaches and even by boastful players, who make exaggerated claims of their ability to track fast shots. Few players are aware of the following salient facts: running causes a remarkable drop in visual acuity; net players often close their eyes when confronted with a high, fast shot; normal blinking reflexes (approximately 16-20 times per minute) cause intermittent, momentary loss of vision; and near-sighted vision, even when corrected by spectacles, is distorted and limited in scope.

The great delusion of tennis, that one can see the ball clearly at all times, is an optical illusion called completion phenomenon. The brain adds clarity when in reality, there is none. From the visual clues it receives from the eyes, the brain completes the trajectory of the ball and seems to keep the ball in focus, even when we are hitting on the run.

VISUAL MEMORY

Vision is a learned experience. It is not automatic. A blind person whose sight is restored by surgery does not instantly see. He cannot recognize objects that in the past he identified by touch. Eventually, he develops a "visual touch," so that a mere glance at an object brings instant recognition.

Much of what happens on a tennis court springs from visual memory. The server keeps his eyes on the ball toss and at no time looks at the court into which he is aiming. The server's target is based on a visual memory of where the court is. In a mindless serve, the ball will either be hit into the net or propelled far too long. Good players study the opponent's court before they hit, to form a strong visual image of court, the net, and the kind of motion they need to clear the net and place a fast ball in the narrow confines of the service court. Eventually, with practice, better players develop "muscle memory." Certain muscle groups respond by rote to a visual memory, and the serve is completed without any conscious effort or visual guidance. In its finest form, the player is like a ball machine, and can spit out balls quite accurately, with robot-like precision. Most players never reach this level of motor memory and hence must rely upon visual memory to control their shots.

Some players have such a strong concept of the court's perimeters that shot-making is automatic. Some tennis players have such a strong visual memory of the tennis court that they imagine they can see and judge their ball's landing position regardless of adverse conditions. This is why professionals frequently argue whether a ball is in or out. At critical times, their strength turns into obstinancy and affects their line calls. Then the player who can find the service court without seeing it and is applauded is greeted by jeers when he calls a ball he did not see and argues with the umpire.

THE SLOW GAME VERSUS THE FAST GAME

Tennis beginners are reared on slow tennis. Easy shots are hit well within their reach and all they are expected to do is to hit them back. Eventually they learn how to stroke the ball and hit while running. The player who has been spoon-fed balls to center court finds it a different game when he has to run. He has to pace himself; he requires earlier preparation for the shot, and he loses a great deal of visual control—running blurs his sight.

The luxury of slow tennis is time. The eyes can see and the body can afford to move leisurely. A full tennis stroke can be made with the arm in preparation, ready for the smooth stroking motion and a complete follow-through. The player is visually secure; he can follow the ball almost to the point of impact.

A slow player cannot compete effectively against a fast player. His eye is trained for the slow shot and his stroke requires more preparation time. Until he learns to cope with speed, the average player cannot expect to improve his game.

Fast tennis heats up the action; consequently, the visual demands are far greater. The player must use a variety of techniques to guide him to the ball, including sound—the sound of his opponent's hit and the sound of the bounce. If there is excessive noise (trains, airplanes, or other) in the vicinity of the court, play is more difficult. There are three basic requirements for fast tennis:

(1) abandoning the trajectory of the oncoming ball

If the player attempts to chase the ball with his eyes, he will be late for every fast shot. The fast ball cannot be followed when it arrives at the edge of a player's field of vision. The faster the ball travels the earlier he loses it.

(2) anticipation

A good player watches the motions of his opponents to anticipate where to run for the return shot. Some players are so skillful, they can judge a shot by their opponent's stroke. The advantage of early anticipation is that the player does not have to see the ball's trajectory as it approaches the hitting zone.

(3) striking the ball early

The player should attempt to hit the ball in front of his body. He never knows the precise position of the ball in relation to the racket. A major fault of players is failing to anticipate the speed of the ball and hitting late. Often there is no time for a full swing.

There is a degree of guesswork to the fast game. There is no time for deliberation. It is a different game with different strokes, and different visual demands.

RUNNING

Running is one of the great spoilers of vision. The point is easily demonstrated. Hold a newspaper in your hand and run in place; your ability to read the print will be impaired. The faster you run, the more your vision is impaired.

Despite the generous size of a tennis ball, good vision is essential because there are so many visual impediments (e.g., running, acceleration, eye movement, illumination, and the speed of the ball).

When a player is running, he may lose sight of a fast ball soon after the opponent makes contact. The ball in flight is seen only as a blur. The better player attempts to eliminate blurred vision by arriving early at the point where he will make contact and stopping before he hits the ball.

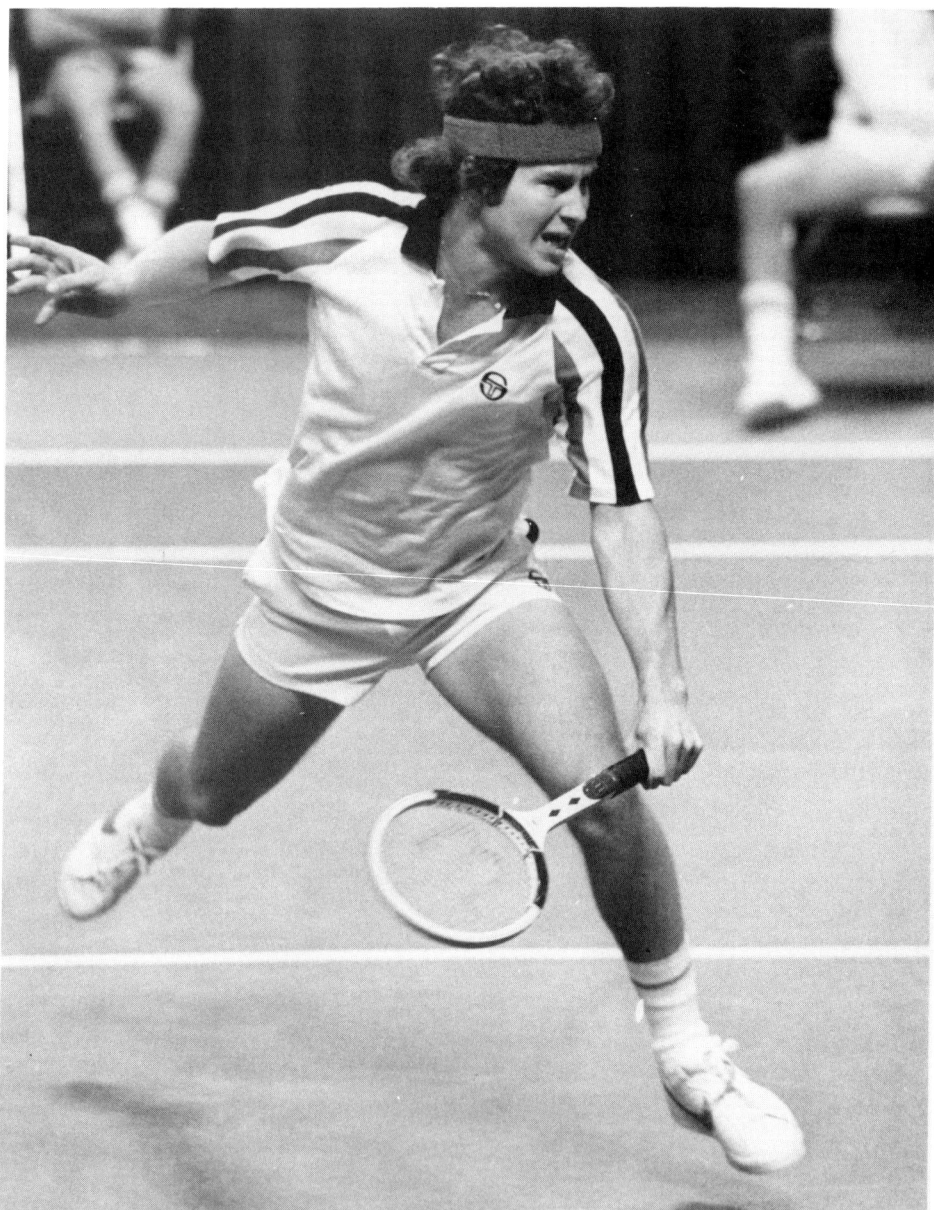

Figure 7-2. John McEnroe running for the ball. The ball is travelling fast; McEnroe is running all-out. (Can a player really accurately assess where a ball hits? We think not.)

There are several styles of running. Some players seem to glide with long smooth strides; although they move quickly, they suffer minimal visual loss. Some players run like a piston, churning up and down. Their body displacement is maximal, resulting in high visual loss. There are even tennis players who run blindly, face to the ground, as if they were doing an intense dash. They have little opportunity to see their opponent hit and cannot adjust properly. And there are variations to these patterns: the slow starter must put forth a great burst of speed to reach the ball, resulting in visual turmoil; the hyperexcitable player charges every ball like a bull going for the cape. He rarely sees the ball clearly and invariably finds himself cramped for a shot because he has run into the hitting zone.

Ideally, a player should run with long, smooth strides, his eyes directed toward the opponent's court. In perfect play, the player is prepared to receive the ball with both feet on the ground so there is little head and body displacement. In reality, most players do well to stop their forward acceleration and keep one foot remaining on the ground. Any reduction of body and head motion improves eyesight.

Fast running may cause vision to drop to the level of legal blindness—the inability to see images at 20 feet that a normal person sees at 200 feet. The tennis player is so accustomed to seeing poorly, he accepts it as the norm.

Good players do not make special visual efforts to play the game. They discover, through trial and error, the proper running speed, acceleration, and timing required to reach the ball in time to stabilize body motion. The cessation of head and body is essential to improving visual performance. Some players have poor running vision. They may hit well against a ball machine or in warm-up practice but perform poorly when forced to run. The best way to improve running vision is to correct running techniques. This can be accomplished effectively through video tapes.

IMPACT—THE BALL STRIKING THE RACKET IS A NONVISUAL EVENT

Only high-speed photography can freeze the moment of impact of a tennis ball on the racket. Many current coaching techniques are predicated on the assumption that the eyes can follow the flight of the ball to impact—an impossibility in the fast game. A player is told to concentrate on the orientation of his racket—is it perpendicular or slanted? He is expected to know: where on the rise of the ball to make contact; where in the arc of the swing to make the hit; and how long a ball will stay on the strings. But, the eyes cannot provide this data, hence they are meaningless coaching techniques.

Some players claim to be able to watch the ball almost to the point of impact. How far away? An inch, perhaps six inches, maybe a foot? Consider the serve: When do you no longer see the ball coming at you—at a distance of three feet, maybe six, or ten? No one is really certain.

Why do their claims of visual control of the ball vary so greatly? The answer has two components: When the ball can be seen is a factor of speed and also of the acuteness of dynamic vision. Dynamic vision depends upon contrast, good illumination, ability to concentrate, and static acuity (the ability to see clearly with the eye at rest). If a player is tired, worried, preoccupied, playing at twilight, or not wearing distance glasses, he will not see the ball early.

It should lift a burden off many tennis students to learn that impact is a nonvisual event. It is certainly a valid goal to try to hit the ball in the middle of the racket, but it is not always possible to succeed. Since many shots are hit "blind," it is wasted effort to worry about the tilt of the racket or the rise of the ball. Photographs of the half volley reveal that players' eyes gaze forward beyond the ball. Their hit is a blind act.

THE PHYSICS OF RACKET SIZE

A player who has only fair dynamic visual acuity should consider seriously using an oversize racket. The physics of oversize rackets have been carefully studied. Dr. Howard Brody, a physicist at the University of Pennsylvania, reported his findings in the *American Journal of Physics*. His research was scholarly and included discussion of percussion centers, vibration nodes, dwell times, asymmetric deflections, and restitution coefficients. He brought to bear the full thrust of a physics laboratory to his tests, employing laser beams, mirrors, and oscilliscopes.

His results were remarkably similar to those of Howard Head, the remarkable man who invented both the Head Ski and the large-size Prince racket. Dr. Brody found that the center of percussion, a vital factor in racket performance, varied from racket to racket. The percussion center is that spot on the racket which, if hit by a ball, will not produce vibration or torque—areas called vibration nodes. If torque occurs, the

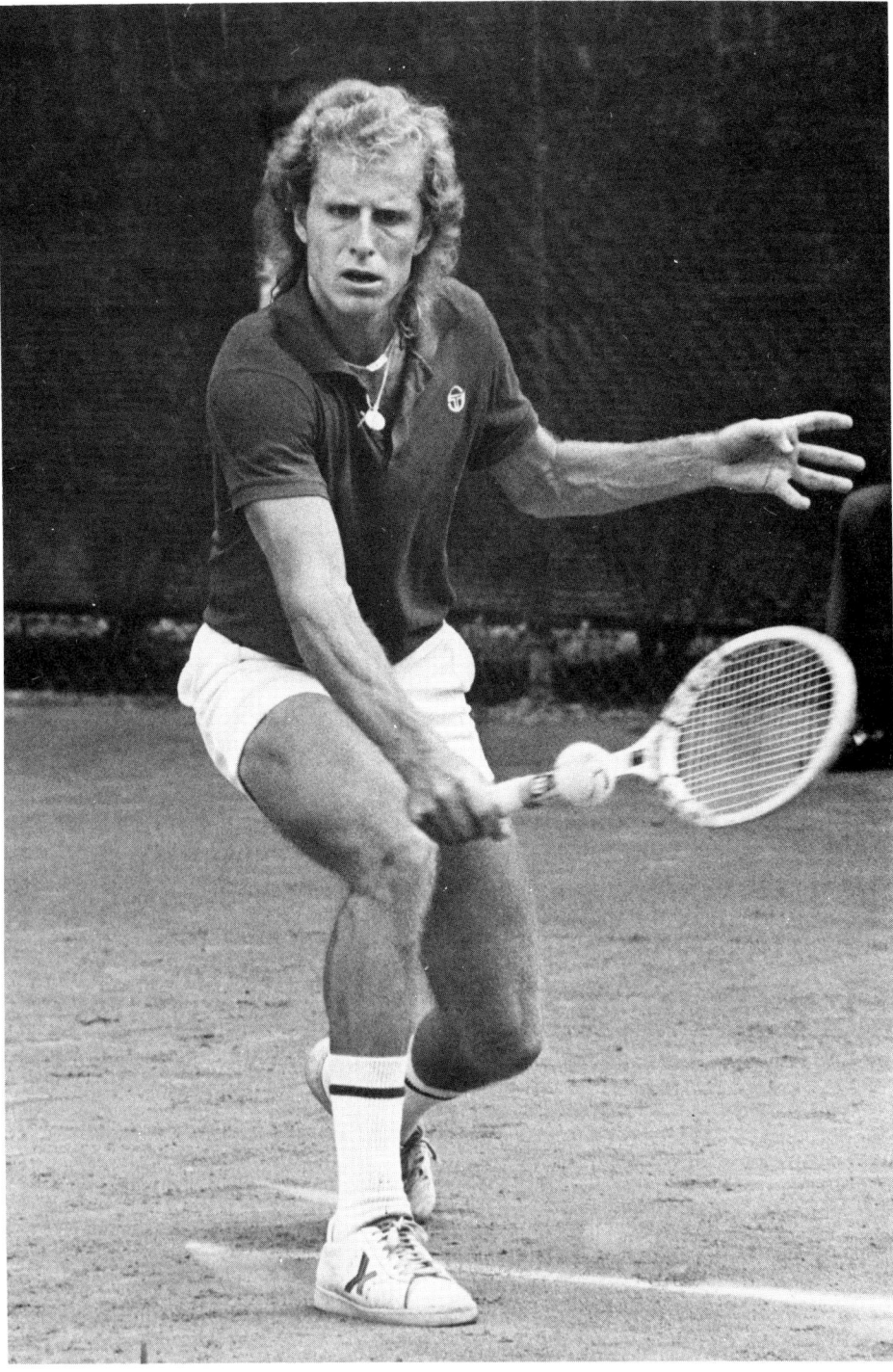

Figure 7-3. Vitas Gerulaitus concentrating but not keeping his eye on the ball.

racket twists in the hand, which strains the muscle of the forearm (one of the principle causes of tennis elbow). Torque also reduces the accuracy of return. The percussion center should be in the center of the racket head, but Dr. Brody found it was an eccentric area, somewhat displaced by an inch or so closer to the handle. In larger rackets, the percussion center is larger and tends to be more centrally placed, with an extension toward the shaft of the racket.

The percussion center is often called the sweet spot, because it is the best place on the racket head to hit a ball. The sweet spot is the center of percussion, the point on the face where impact produced no vibration at the end of the handle.

If the ball strikes the racket on a line perpendicular to it, the ball will rebound straight or at a 180-degree line. But if the ball hits the racket at an off-center point, the ball will rebound at an angle. The farther from the sweet spot the ball makes contact with the racket, the farther askew it will go. Thus the direction of the ball coming off the racket can be changed radically according to the place on the racket head the ball is hit. The path of the returned ball does not depend solely on position of impact on the racket but also on the inclination of the racket. If the racket head is tilted back at impact, the ball will rise and tend to go forward and up; if it is tilted down, the ball will head into the net. Ideally then, the ball should strike the sweet spot at the moment the racket is vertical. As we have said, it is not possible to see this happen, but the player should keep a strong grip to prevent tilting caused by the force of the ball.

Dr. Brody also found that the energy of the oncoming ball is not radically dissipated by its collision with the gut or nylon of the racket. The distance of the ball's rebound is determined by its coefficient of restitution. This is the ratio of velocity after collision to the velocity before collision. He found that the kinetic energy of the tennis ball is diminished by only a half with impact. Howard Head also studied the coefficient of restitution and discovered that the return velocity of a ball struck at an area outside the sweet spot could be one-third to one-half the velocity of a ball struck in the sweet spot. Moreover, on his own Prince racket, he found a very high-velocity-return area close to the throat of the racket that was not present on other tennis rackets. This meant that not only was direction of the ball more accurate after hitting the sweet spot, but the force of return power was greater.

In effect, when the center of percussion and the center of the racket coincide, the resultant shot produces the least vibration.

Dr. Brody, using a laser beam, measured the duration of impact and found it was only five milliseconds. This incredibly short interval does not permit the eye to see what is happening. The time cycle is slightly greater if one includes the total time for the racket head to bend back when hit by the ball and return to its normal position. The dwell time — the time that the ball stays in contact with the gut — is shortened, however, if the racket is strung tighter.

Most of the events at impact require laser beams or strobe photography to detail the action. Since impact cannot be seen, it makes sense to use a racket with a larger sweet spot for optimum hitting power and control of the ball. Great players do not need the benefit of the larger surface as much as average or club players. The professionals and top amateurs have the anticipation, the fast moves, the sharpness of excellent dynamic acuity, and the proper strokes to insure that the ball will be returned effectively. The intermediate players, while playing the fast game, are frequently unable to cope with the demands of accelerated hitting time. They hit while running; they fail to read the signals of their opponent's next shot correctly; and they move without proper timing, resulting in awkward body positions (totally outstretched or uncomfortably cramped). They don't have the conditioning or coordination to deal with the demands of accelerated tennis. The larger racket does not correct the essential faults in the player's game but it increases the odds that the sweet spot will be hit.

TENNIS INJURIES — SINGLES AND DOUBLES

Tennis injuries are more likely to occur when the velocity of the ball is maximum and its trajectory is towards the eye. Both conditions are encountered at the net. The pace of the ball has not been dissipated by flight or by bounce, and it often crosses the net at eye level. It is rare for the ball to ricochet off a racket and strike the eye — we have never witnessed such mishap. Clinically, the jeopardy of tennis is at the net.

Net play occurs in either singles or doubles. The singles player must move quickly to net with a smooth, gliding motion to avoid blurring his vision of the opponent and the ball. He must maintain a balance between clear vision and running fast enough to arrive at net before or during the opponent's swing. Coming off a serve is an ideal time, when momentum is carrying the body forward. The opponent is forced to remain in the back court and will often hit a return. Although serve and volley game creates an ideal opportunity for eye injuries, in fact, they occur infrequently. Among the 20 top-ranked professionals, an eye injury in singles play has not been reported in the past 5 years. The low injury rate among top-ranked players is attributable to their excellent anticipation of the ball and good reflexes. The club player is spared eye injury because most returns of service are weak block shots with no pace on the ball. Because of the low incidence of injury, eye protection devices are not indicated or warranted for singles tennis.

Eye injury is most likely to occur in doubles. The action of the game is always directed towards the net, with the players pressing forward for blanket coverage of the net. The rhythmical cadence of the base line player in singles is replaced by the choppy, karate-style motions of the doubles players volleying at the net. The jeopardy is enhanced by the fast play, in which successive volleys may never touch the ground. The ball may be returned high at eye level. The jeopardy is so real that many club players, in critical situations, will raise their rackets in front of their face for protection.

The players who shield their face with their rackets to avoid injury cannot play an effective net game. They should wear eye protection.

Eye injuries are more common with:

(a) The novice — their skills of anticipation are poor. Their opponents are often new players also, who frequently play in a clumsy or erratic fashion. The ball may be returned as slowly as a falling leaf or it may be bashed forward as though fired from a cannon. The novice on the receiving end, if he sees the ball at all, has to protect his face.

(b) The elderly — it is quite common for players between 50 to 60 years old to stop playing singles and retire to doubles. They have the skills to make a shot but not the legs to run for the ball. The level of their game is high, their shots strong and accurate, but they may lack the agility to deflect a shot or protect their face when the need arises. The singles game they can no longer play was actually safer.

(c) The very skilled doubles player who aggressively attacks the net all the time. These players are strong athletes with the coordination, fitness, experience and expertise to play the game at its highest level. The velocity of the ball is frequently over 100 miles an hour — too fast even for these strong, responsive athletes to visually control the play all the time. Such players are usually fearless with regard to the dangers offered by a tennis ball.

(d) The sadist who takes positive glee in intimidating his opponent by hitting the ball as hard as possible. The ball is used as a weapon of fear to unsettle the opponent. It is unpleasant tennis, but played by all types of people.

(e) The masochist — simply stands there when the ball is blasted his way. He seems to want to be injured and often gets his wish.

In our records, we have found 11 cases of tennis-related injuries. The types of injury include:

Retinal Detachment	2 cases
Hyphema	4 cases (Associated with hyphema was recession of the angle structures, iris dialysis and rupture of the sphincter muscle.)
Contusion of the Lids	3 cases
Macular Edema	3 cases (Both cases of retinal detachment also had macular edema.)
Iritis	3 cases (Two of these cases had contusion of the lids as well. Although infrequent, injuries are apt to be serious when they occur.)
Loss of Vision	4 cases (20/40 became 20/100)
Excessive Photophopia	4 cases (Due to rupture of the sphincter muscle of the iris. The affected pupil was fixed and semi-dilated.)
Unilateral Glaucoma	2 cases (Occurred 4 years after the eye injury. One patient initially had a hyphema and one initially presented with iritis. There was also a partial subluxation of the lens.)
Cataract	1 case (Occurred 3 years after the injury.)

Of this group, 8 of the 11 injuries occurred during doubles play, and only 3 occurred during singles. In each case, injury could have been prevented with the use of 3 mm thick polycarbonate lenses.

The actual frequency of injury is probably higher, but many cases are not reported. The tennis ball is large as opposed to a squash ball. A tennis ball is likely to be stopped by the frontal bone, the nasal bones, or the malar bone. Unlike a squash ball, which is harder and smaller, a tennis ball does not easily fit into the orbital recess, the concavity in which the eye itself rests. Thus most injuries cause direct contusion of the lids, which become swollen, with or without ecchymosis. If the injury is severe, there may be secondary contusion to the eye itself.

The incidence of injuries is probably too low to recommend mandatory safety glasses for tennis players. No large series of tennis eye injuries has ever been reported. Safety glasses should be considered in special instances: in doubles play involving the elderly, the novice, and players who play aggressively.

Despite the relative softness of a tennis ball, its velocity can exceed 100 miles an hour. Serious injuries, with loss of vision, do occur.

SAFETY PRECAUTIONS

People who normally wear glasses should get special safety glasses that are chemically or heat hardened. They must be at least 3.0 mm thick to be able to withstand the impact of a one-inch steel ball dropped from a height of 50 inches. Plastic lenses must be specially designed to withstand the same tests. The best plastic is polycarbonate, which can withstand the impact of a bullet without shattering. Flexible nylon frames that have a cushioned rubber bridge are a good choice, because the frames can be adjusted for comfort and will not snap if hit.

There are plastic guards available now, which can be used for tennis and squash, or racquetball. These are made of shatterproof plastic and are transparent allowing the wearer wide peripheral vision. These protectors are form-fitting, comfortable, and completely protect the eye. The "combat" glasses are among the best of these plastic guards.

Eye protection is now becoming commonplace. For years it has been mandatory in industry, and is now required for amateur hockey. Eye safety is actively promoted in squash and racquetball, both of which have a high incidence of ocular injury.

Tennis is a little different from other racket sports. The ball is large and relatively soft; the racket is large and can guard the face. Deflections from the net come up to the face without speed and are of inconsequential danger. Orthopedic surgeons seem to see the greatest number of tennis injuries, those that are endemic to the sport—torn knee ligaments and cartilages and bad backs.

Eye injuries, though infrequent, tend to be serious when they occur. In high-risk situations, always wear protective lenses.

COURT SURFACES

There are many court surfaces. Each has its characteristics, which must be understood. To play effectively, players must learn to modify their game to suit each type of surface. At one end of the scale are clay and synthetic courts, which can be extremely slow; at the opposite end are cement and grass courts which are fast.

Clay Courts

Clay courts give the game an easy cadence and impart a gentleness that is tennis tradition. It is very comfortable on the feet, as the player slides easily into each stroke. The sound of the ball is muffled, in contrast to the sharp crack of an asphalt return. The court's clay surface slows the ball.

Clay-type courts have a top surface that is made of granular crushed stone or brick. In Europe, brick is frequently used, and the courts are often a red color. In the eastern United States, clay is a common court surface because of the abundance of crushed gravel. The color is a neutral gray. Clay courts suffer, because they need constant attention. The surface is soft and loose and requires watering to hold it and compacting by roller to keep it even.

The bounce off a clay court is relatively slow and high. The hitter may find it difficult to put shots out of reach of a good retriever. Thus the rallies tend to be long and demanding but strokes are often relaxed.

Clay courts demand a certain strategy. The net must not be rushed with abandon. The high bounce gives a player sufficient time to reach and see the ball, and the man at the net may be passed either on the sides or with a lob. Clay court play is essentially a baseline game, where steadiness is a greater asset than hitting the ball fast. Volleys must be well placed and solidly hit or the balls can be returned. The service ace loses its sizzle once it hits the clay surface. Hence, most players rely on spins and accurate placement for a more effective serve.

Cement Courts

The pace of the ball off a cement court is very fast. The clay court player will find his game shattered by the demands of the fast ball. Everything is accelerated. The ball cannot be seen or followed so it must be hit early; the time to reach the ball is reduced, so that the play must be anticipated earlier, the running accelerated, and the motion of the stroke either speeded up or abbreviated. Points are quickly made because it is easier to put the ball away. The diligent clay court retriever is invariably the loser on cement, the surface preferred by flashier players.

Cement is the hardest surface. The ball loses little speed on the bounce; it bounces well but not as high as on clay. Some courts have a cement base with a textured top layer to make the game more comfortable for the legs and the feet. The top layers of cement courts have widely differing characteristics, which effect the bounce of the ball.

The type of game played is determined by the surface characteristics and the nature of the bounce. Among the professionals, there are surface specialists. Chris Evert's winning streak on clay is the stuff of legends, while Roscoe Tanner's serve and volley game is more suited to a hard surface. Occasionally a player, like Bjorn Borg, plays well on all of them. Paradoxically, Borg uses a baseline, clay-court strategy to win on fast courts. He can keep his eyes on the ball longer than players who repeatedly dash aggressively to net. To accomplish this feat and return an offensive ball, he anticipates well and moves quickly. The fast cement court favors the player with a cannonball serve. The ball travels too quickly for the eye to follow. The opponent has little reflex time and must play with a stiffer wrist, a shorter backswing, and greater forward movement into the ball. Many professionals, such as Arthur Ashe, advise merely getting the ball back, even at the risk of set-up. On cement, a spin serve can be devastating, because in addition to its speed the ball may hop to the right or left.

Cement is a demanding and punishing surface. It can get very hot; it is uncomfortable for the legs; and the fast game creates extra stress on the eyes. Asphalt is a little slower than concrete, but it still favors the aggressive player.

Cement is a poor choice for players over forty, for players who do not have perfect vision, and for players who are slow runners or lack physical fitness. These people will derive greater enjoyment from playing on clay.

Grass

Grass is still the surface of champions and is where the roots of tennis lie. As long as Wimbledon remains the world premier tennis tournament, grass remains important for the professional. For the club player, grass is a historical curio, a touch of old England, tea, strawberries and cream, and the pomp of the old Empire.

Visually, grass is a treat—the color green is relaxing and easy on the eye. It offers good contrast under a variety of lighting conditions. Unlike red clay, which can add stress to a nervous player's game, grass relaxes the anxious player.

Grass is a fast surface. The ball bounces lower than on any other surface and it may slide, which makes judgment difficult. The best grass courts are not absolutely smooth or even, and erratic bounces must be anticipated.

The professionals have to constantly adapt their game and gear up for the most demanding surface of all — the Wimbledon grass. It is a totally different experience as it challenges the player's wits and visual prowess to the limit.

Grass is not especially popular in regular tennis play. It is expensive to install and maintain in perfect condition. It taxes the tennis player's skills to the utmost. It deserves to be special.

POINTERS ON COURT SURFACES

(1) It is a good practice to adjust the racket strings to suit the surface. A racket strung with loose tension gives better control on clay surfaces. For fast surface courts, such as cement or grass, a more tightly strung racket will ensure a maximum ball velocity. Most professionals string their rackets between 60 and 65 pounds per square inch to gain extra power. A good club player will string his racket to a pressure of 55 pounds per square inch. The more tightly the racket is strung, the greater the force of the rebound. A very taut racket is like playing with a board — it has no "give," and the shot is harder to control. Bjorn Borg, who has all the talent a tennis player could want, strings his racket to 80 pounds per square inch. Even among professionals, such string tension is exceptionally stiff.

(2) Adjustment to a new surface requires a change of timing to suit the height and speed of ball. In making the transition from one court surface to another, remember to always take the racket back as early as possible to avoid rushing the stroke.

(3) Try to play on a surface that is commensurate with your ability. The best surface is the one you play on the most. It is difficult to adjust one's game to a variety of court surfaces. Club players who attempt it never really acquire any facility in their game, because they must constantly adapt to the variability of the speed of the ball. They never learn to adjust their strokes to a given velocity, hence their timing is off.

A player who constantly loses on concrete may become a winner on clay. The visual adaptation is easier from fast to slow courts, which allows strokes to become long and flowing. The fastest road to improvement is to put the game in slow motion — find a slower tennis surface.

INDOOR VERSUS OUTDOOR TENNIS

Anyone who has played all winter on a tennis court indoors will find that his game seems to have deteriorated when he goes outdoors again. Various conditions contribute to the difficulties of outdoor play:

(1) Wind

Crosswinds, headwinds, and tailwinds alternately slow and speed the ball or propel it out of reach, confusing a player's timing and stroke mechanics.

(2) Sun

Sunlight greatly improves vision. Sunlight causes pupillary constriction, increasing the depth of focus and visibility while running. Spatial judgments will be altered because of pupillary constriction. One's judgment of the ball in flight will be slightly different outdoors than indoors. Although visual conditions are better, errors are made initially, because the eye is not accustomed to the improved lighting.

(3) Physical ground clues

Spatial localization of the ball is easier indoors, where the ceiling, walls, and lights provide orientation for tracking the flight of the ball. The sense of unlimited, free space outdoors reduces the player's auditory and visual clues to the ball's location—even clouds help the player locate the ball. Perhaps the only advantage of outdoor play is that the height of the lob is not limited by a ceiling.

(4) Colors and vision

Accommodation to light and space is not easy. Light adds a feeling of space—white expands space. Typically, the player who moves to an outdoor court hits his ball long or runs into the ball, because he misjudges the distance. It takes anywhere from one to two weeks to make the adjustment to the new space. To test the visual effects of light on space look at a white square on a black background, and then a black square on a white background, both squares having identical measurements. The white square will give the illusion of being larger.

Some players use the sun to their advantage and lob the ball to their opponent who is facing into the sun. As a tactic, it is no worse than hitting the ball to the opponent's weak backhand and an accepted part of the game. The best antidote to blinding sun is sunglasses.

Although indoor tennis does provide almost perfect conditions, most players prefer the aesthetics of playing outdoors in good weather.

WIND, SUN, AND SPACE

Allowance must be made for the wind factor. Its strength and direction will affect play strategy. If the wind is blowing into your back, it is good strategy to hit low topspin groundstrokes, spin serves, and passing shots rather than lobs. If you are facing the wind, it is advisable to hit hard, flat groundstrokes and serves and to hit lobs rather than passing shots. If the wind is blowing across the court, care must be taken to keep the ball from blowing.

If the wind blows the ball after the bounce, it is difficult to change one's mental plan and body motion. Fortunately, the racket is large and may still contact the ball, but probably not the best part.

Bright sunlight creates glare and even temporary blindness. At times, the ball is painful to see. This condition results from the sudden, intense pupillary constriction when looking into the sun. Heavily tinted sunglasses (gray shades are best) should be used for serving into the sun.

Problems of spatial orientation may occur when a player shifts from day to night play. Night tennis causes an expansion of the court, because the illuminated court becomes a white rectangle with a black background, and reference points above and nearby are lost in the darkness. Even the professionals do not like night play.

Perhaps the best solution for ball control in extended space is to use topspin. Topspin is imparted by a racket that travels from a relatively low backswing position and ends in a high follow-through. This results in a higher air pressure on the top of the ball, forcing the ball down. Thus the ball can be hit with considerable power and still stay in the court.

LINE DISPUTES

Line disputes are the bane of the temperamental player. For the professional, one bad call can throw off his game and cost him the set, his earnings, and his rank. Ilie Nastase is reknowned for his temperamental blow-ups over disputed line calls. His theatrical tantrums are reputed to be part show but also outrage that he has not been treated fairly by the umpire. His rage became so intense in a recent major Toronto tournament that he was thrown out of the match and forfeited the largest tennis prize to date. John McEnroe was dubbed "superbrat" by the British media for his emotional outbursts over line calls. A reformed Jimmy Connors is more contained, but his anger is still visible if a call displeases him.

Arguments over line calls are not limited to professionals. It is an unspoken controversy in the average club game. Why unspoken? Because tennis still clings to its Wimbledon heritage of being a gentleman's game. Hard feelings do occur but usually are suppressed; it is considered bad tennis etiquette to vent hostile feelings during a tennis match.

Line-call disputes arise, because everyone believes in the infallibility of their senses, especially their eyes. "I saw it with my own eyes" is a statement that accepts no compromise. One can hedge on a belief or an interpretation but not on a sensory experience. Most people trust their eyes and will fault the opponent, who stands to gain from falsifying the call. If the disagreement calls are numerous, anger may surface into open hostility. Some players deport themselves more professionally than others.

In reality, no player is able to see all the shots of a tennis game. If you are tired or not concentrating when a fast service lands in your court, there is a distinct possibility you will not see the bounce, even miss it entirely. If you are moving, vision is further compromised so there is a better than average chance that you won't clearly see a ball played near the line.

A player's ability to call the shot depends upon the speed of the ball, his body motion, and his visual acuity. Eyesight also depends on such variables as correct eyeglasses, color of the ball, and light conditions.

In professional tennis, the best eyes belong to the referee. Most of the action occurs within his fixed visual field. Furthermore, the referee does not have any bias to color his perceptions. Despite these advantages, the referee is not infallible, but he should be given the benefit of doubt. He is in a far better position to make a visual judgment.

For the majority of us who do not play with a referee on hand, there are some basic conventions to help determine line calls.

Rule #1: The stationary player is in the best position to make a line call. In doubles, it may be oneself or one's opponent standing at the net. In singles, the matter is more difficult to resolve. If both players are in motion and the action is fast, neither player can see the ball clearly. On the service if there is a disagreement over the call, the service should be taken over, because neither player can make a sound judgment. However, if the server does not run to net, visual advantage belongs to him. His body and head are still permitting him to watch the trajectory of the ball. The opponent closest to the ball has to move to pick up a high velocity missile. His visual abilities are not adequate for the task.

Rule #2: In slow tennis, the player closest to the bounce is in best position to judge the line call. This is particularly true of baseline shots.

Rule #3: In fast tennis if both players are in motion, the play should be repeated if there is controversy. The most courteous players will give the point to their opponent to eliminate the bitterness of line disputes.

Rule #4: If there is any doubt about the call, give the advantage to your opponent. The win-loss ratio of points is the same whether players are mutually courteous or mutually hostile.

Calling line shots is one of the most controversial subjects in tennis. It adversely affects professional play, club play, and can even spoil a harmless game among children. Line disputes can be settled only when players recognize the limitations and fallibility of their dynamic visual acuity.

In recent years, an electronic field has been set up at Wimbledon and the United States Open to aid the linesmen. The referees and linesmen are taught not to follow the ball, but rather to look intently at the lines keeping their head and eyes absolutely still. Yet occasionally they do make errors and for especially human reasons—blinking just as the ball bounces. The electronic monitor is perhaps the best way to make accurate calls.

GLASSES, SUNGLASSES, AND CONTACT LENSES

Most people who wear glasses occasionally (for driving or movies) will also wear them for playing tennis. Others, however, prefer slight reduction in vision to the nuisance of wearing glasses. Do the advantages of wearing glasses outweigh the disadvantages? It must be an individual decision, largely dependent upon such factors as personal comfort and the degree and type of refractive error.

Individuals with myopia or astigmatism, no matter how mild the error, may require glasses to avoid eye strain and headache.

Most ophthalmologists agree that glasses (especially in high powers to correct large refractive errors) make it difficult to play superb tennis. There are so many disadvantages (e.g., vision obscured by fogging and perspiration, glare), glasses must be considered a burden.

In view of how many professionals wear glasses quite successfully, however, glasses cannot be considered a handicap for the tennis athlete. Arthur Ashe frequently alternates between glasses and contact lenses.

Billy Jean King wears glasses all the time, and now Martina Navratilova, as well, wears glasses for tournaments.

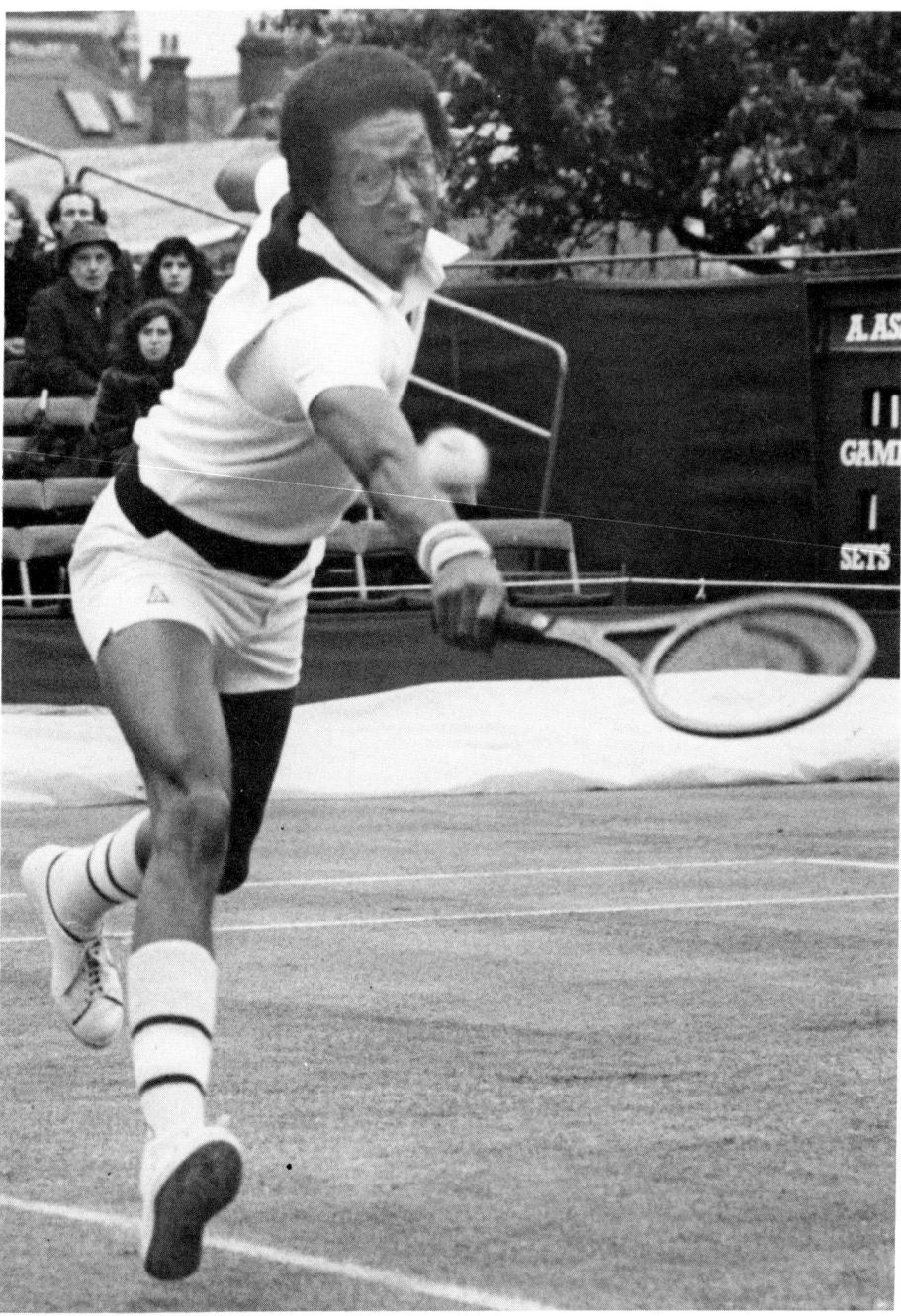

Figure 7-4. Arthur Ashe alternates between glasses and contact lenses.

In borderline cases, where glasses may not make a great deal of difference, it is useful to remember that perfect optics are not possible in tennis, where running decreases vision from 20/20 to 20/60 or 20/70. What is lacking in resolution and clarity can be made up in anticipation.

SUMMARY

(1) Start quickly but run slowly (and smoothly) to meet the ball. Try to reach the ball with at least one foot stable to ensure optimum visual stability for maximum power and control of the ball. When the body is in motion, there can be no body stability to leverage a shot, and vision is greatly reduced. The faster the run, the worse the vision. Good players seem to glide.

(2) Tailor the stroke shot to the speed of the ball. The faster the ball is traveling, the more imperative it is to hit in front of the body. Anticipate early and move into the trajectory of the ball. Many club players experience no growth or maturity in their tennis development because their game is too rigid. Their motor memory is geared to the slow game. Such players, who cannot change their ingrained visual habits, should try to slow down the game by hitting lobs and medium-paced shots to the baseline.

(3) Oversize racket — asset or liability: The aerodynamics of a large and small racket may be the same but in clinical tests of the oversize racket, most players found it lacking in maneuverability. An oversize racket is excellent in doubles, where fast net play is paramount. A volley shot is one of the fastest shots in tennis, and a bigger racket compensates for the visual loss. It is not helpful where the service is derived from a snap of the wrist.

(4) Anticipation is the antidote to blurred vision. Some players try to gain visual advantage by avoiding the net and receiving service far behind the baseline. But the visual gains are lost by the necessity to run farther (laterally) and faster to reach the ball.

(5) Develop visual memory for serving. The server should look at the opponent's service court just before he tosses a ball. He then hits blind, his arm guided by a visual memory of the target etched in his mind just prior to the toss. The toss must become mechanical so he is free to concentrate on the visual memory.

(6) Good depth perception is important for net play and volley shots. Accurate depth perception requires equal vision in both eyes. One good

eye cannot do the job of two eyes. The lob shot moving in space is difficult and requires good depth perception. To receive the lob, point at the ball with your free hand, keeping the racket in the back scratch position as when serving. The lob ball drops quickly (the service ball is hit at almost zero velocity) and must be hit earlier and higher if a smash shot is intended. The speed of the racket determines the visual complexity of the shot. A smash is more difficult, because a fast-falling ball is met by a fast racket and the area of impact is blurred. If the ball is hit slowly, the visual hold on the ball is longer and the shot is apt to be more precise. Concentrate on placing the overhead smash; develop accuracy and gradually add the power. The player with poor depth perception should allow the ball to bounce.

(7) One of the most difficult shots to make is the half volley, a forced stroke, executed when the ball lands at your feet during a rush to net. It is a totally blind hit. Even the bounce is not seen. The ratio of anticipation to vision is 100 percent anticipation and zero vision. The half volley shot has neither power nor placement. The racket must be open-faced to force the ball to clear the net, and the player must get down to the ball, so the return will not be an easy put-away for the opponent.

(8) Lines calls are subject to all the inaccuracies of our vision, caused by motion, poor depth perception, and eye glasses. The courteous player understands the fallibility of his eyesight and awards the point to his opponent or asks for a replay of the point. Tennis should relieve tension rather than create it.

(9) The net game should be an integral part of every warm-up to avoid the menace response (i.e., automatic closure of the eyelid to any stimulus that threatens the eye). Many players at net close their eyes when they see a fast tennis ball coming. The lid closure is involuntary and prolonged; it is not a blink. The player is not aware he does it. The only way to control the reaction is to practice volley shots at the net. Once the eyes are not threatened by the ball, they will stay open. Once a player feels comfortable at the net, he can once again use his racket as intended, to play tennis, rather than as a facial protector.

(10) Be aware of the common symptoms of sensory fatigue and/or lack of physical fitness:

— Seeing the ball late — there does not seem to be enough time to get the racket back.
— Loss of concentration; difficulty following the ball; player unconsciously moves back to take a slower ball.

— Player complains about the lighting. It seems darker and dynamic visual acuity requires contrast.
— Player begins to make gross line-call errors.
— Player is less inclined to head for the net.
— Difficulty with return of service; faulty anticipation because opponent is not seen clearly.
— Inaccurate estimates of ball speed resulting in need to run faster.
— Player loses competitive edge after only 30 minutes of singles play, and his game deteriorates.

What can be done to combat these debilitating symptoms? Aerobic fitness is the key. The eyes are like a camera taking pictures, which are then relayed to the occipital cortex, the visual area of the brain. When the oxygen supply to the brain is reduced, the light sensitivity of the brain is depressed, causing a pronounced darkening effect. A good tennis player should be a good athlete.

REFERENCES

1. Bard, C., Fleury, M.: Analysis of visual search activity during sport problem situations. *J Hum Mov St 3:* 214, 1976.
2. Hoffman, L.G., Rouse, M., Ryan, J.B.: Dynamic visual acuity: A review. *Am Optom Assoc 52:* 833, 1981.
3. Ditchburn, R., Binsborg, B.: Vision with stabilized retinal image. *Nature 170:* 36, 1952.
4. Ditchburn, R., Fender, D., Mayne, S.: Vision with controlled movements of the retinal image. *Physiol 145:* 98, 1959.
5. Hoshikawa, H., Takahashi, M., Fujishiro, T., Midorikawa, C.: Gaze stabilization during stepping and running. *Nippon Jibiinkoka Gakhai Kaiko 86:* 881, 1983.
6. Daroff, R.B.: Physiologic anatomic and pathophysiologic considerations of eye movements. *Trans Opthalmol Soc UK 90:* 409, 1970.
7. Duke, M.: Tennis players and eye injuries. *JAMA 236:* 2287, 1976.
8. Easterbrook, W.M.: Eye injuries in racquet sports: A continuing problem. *Can Med Assoc J 123:* 268, 1980.
9. Holter, N.: Tennis balls and eye injuries. *JAMA 237:* 1312, 1977.
10. Ramanan, S.: Eye injuries from tennis balls. *JAMA 236:* 1355, 1976.
11. Vinger, P.F.: Sports-related eye injury: A preventable problem. *Surv Ophthalmol 25:* 47, 1980.
12. Vinger, P.F., Tolpin, D.W.: Racquet sports: An ocular hazard. *JAMA 239:* 2575, 1978.

CHAPTER 8

AVIATION OPHTHALMOLOGY

WAYNE WHITMORE

AVIATION IS, traditionally, a practical means of transportation. However, flying, whether it be in a fixed wing aircraft or rotorcraft, can also be pursued for sport. Flying a glider, ultralight, or a balloon certainly should be considered a sport, along with aerobatics (stunt flying) and aircraft racing. A pilot may be challenged both physically and mentally during these types of flight. Controlling an aircraft requires concentration, coordination, timing, judgment and, most importantly, good vision.

Aircraft racing became a pure sporting activity after World War II. Prior to that time it was considered an arena for the testing of new aircraft design and the improvement of aircraft performance. Racing pilots were military pilots or professionals, subsidized by commercial industry or by the government, to fly expensive aircraft which individuals could not afford to maintain. Now, with the advent of class racing, aircraft of equal performance characteristics and within the economic capabilities of the general public, can be flown in competition. These events are, primarily a test of pilot skill and not a comparison of the power or maneuverability of one aircraft over another.

Aerobatics have been performed ever since aircraft were built to withstand the forces of the maneuvers (and sometimes when they were not). Aerobatics probably represent the biggest challenge to pilots because of the disorienting accelerative forces the pilot is subjected to. There are now many competitions throughout the country (and the world) for aircraft racing of both low and high performance aircraft, and aerobatics on several different levels.

Without a doubt, vision is the most important sense when flying an aircraft. To emphasize this point, it need only be realized that when flying without visual reference to the surrounding conditions (fog or clouds) and to the instruments in the aircraft, it cannot be determined which direction is up or down. Without instruments or outside visual references, it is only through acceleration or deceleration that the vestibular system of the inner ear can perceive a change in motion. This system is not sensitive enough to detect subtle control changes (above aircraft vibrations) which could quickly cause a pilot to lose control of his aircraft. On terra firma, where travel is in two dimensions and the accelerative forces are less complicated, the constant pull of gravity tells us which direction is up or down. When flying an aircraft, movement is three dimensional. The forces can be changed so that an accelerative force through the vertical axis of the aircraft which is greater than, less than, or equal to that of gravity may be directed at an angle other than 90 degrees to the earth's surface. For example, in a balanced 60 degree bank turn where the aircraft is maintaining a constant altitude, a force twice that of gravity (2 G), is exerted by the pilot and passengers on their seats at an angle of 30 degrees to the earth's surface. Vision is the quintessential sense allowing pilots to recover safely from their aerobatic maneuvers and to turn, while racing at several hundred miles per hour, around a pylon a handful of yards away. Without vision, there is no flying.

AVIATION REGULATIONS

The United States government has, fortunately, seen fit to create the Federal Aviation Regulations (FAR) which govern all aspects of flying, from the construction and maintenance of aircraft, to the training and physical requirements of pilots. The medical requirements are set down in the FARs part 67. The visual requirements (Appendix I) differ slightly (as do the other medical requirements) for the three classes of medical certificates. These certificates permit a pilot to fly aircraft for certain purposes, if he has the appropriate training requirements and/or license. Several of the requirements are ambiguous, leaving it up to the examiner (based on his understanding of the visual tasks required to fly safely) to determine whether or not the person being examined is qualified. A medical certificate is not required to fly a glider or an ultralight aircraft, allowing the pilot himself to be the judge of his physical capability to fly.

The first and second class medical certificates entitle a pilot with the appropriate license and ratings to fly commercial aircraft which are used for hire, or to carry passengers for profit. Most commercial airlines in the United States, including all of the larger ones, require an airline transport pilot (ATP) license for their crew. This license may only be obtained if one has a first-class medical certificate. In order to remain active, this certificate must be renewed every six months. The second-class medical certificate is slightly less rigid than the first-class in its requirements, and is valid for one year. The third-class certificate, good for two years, is significantly less rigid in its requirements than the previous two. Pilots with third-class certificates are not permitted to fly passengers or cargo for hire, but may use their aircraft to carry passengers for recreation or business where money is made directly by using the aircraft.

When making application for any of the three medical certificates, both glasses and contact lenses may be used to fulfill the requirements. A visual acuity of 20/20 or better in each eye, with or without correction, is required while flying an aircraft commercially. The pilot's uncorrected acuity cannot be less than 20/100 in either eye. For recreational flying, under a third-class medical certificate, a visual acuity of 20/50 or better in each eye without correction is permitted. However, if the acuity is less than this in one eye, the visual acuity must be corrected to 20/30 or better in each eye. This means that someone whose best vision is 20/40 in each eye with correction (and less than 20/50 in one eye without correction), is not eligible for this medical certificate. Conversely, an individual with uncorrected vision of 20/50 in each eye, will still be eligible for a third-class license, even though his vision can not be improved with the use of corrective lenses. The logic behind this regulation is questionable, but then, many government regulations can be considered illogical.

Near vision, with the appropriate presbyopic add in the glasses sufficient to read aviation maps in dim light, is essential for commercial pilots applying for first and second-class certificates. There is no near vision requirement for a third-class medical certificate, and if the presbyopic pilot who forgets his glasses wants some accurate navigational information from his maps, he must ask his fearless passengers. The ability to distinguish red, green, and white signals is a requirement for all classes of medical certificates, since these are the signals used at controlled airports to direct traffic (in the air and on the ground) in case of radio communications failure.

Normal visual fields are required for a commercial license and pilots flying commercially are not permitted to have any eye disease. The third-class certificate allows mild eye disease ("no serious eye pathology") and makes no specific mention of visual fields. Binocularity with small amounts of heterophoria is permitted for the commercial pilots, provided there is not a breakdown in fusion under flight conditions. There is no requirement for binocularity in the third-class medical certificate, which is surprising considering the importance of having some degree of stereopsis to determine distances, especially when taking off or landing an aircraft. Obviously, the medical examiner must use his discretion when deciding whether or not a certain visual handicap amounts to a hazard for the pilot and his possible passengers, not to mention the people on the ground.

SITUATIONAL LIGHTING AND OPTICAL ILLUSIONS

Having good visual function, and using it in an effective way while flying, are entirely different. Experience and training are as important to visual function while flying as they are to the actual flying itself. An experienced pilot will scan the horizon from the cockpit searching for other aircraft, stopping his eyes at various points to allow his peripheral vision to detect movement while the eyes are fixed. The eyes cannot detect the fine movements of distant aircraft in their peripheral visual fields if they themselves are moving.

Glare, a consequence of light scattering within the eye, leads to a reduction in contrast of the retinal image and, hence, visual acuity. This condition is thought to be caused by the excessive bleaching of the retinal photopigments and diffraction caused by too small a pupil. A pilot should, therefore, avoid situations where he is flying into the sun, where he is subjected to sunlight shining off bodies of water, or where reflections are caused by sunlight striking the slick surfaces of the aircraft. To prevent pilot fatigue due to squinting, the use of filters is recommended for prolonged flight in bright environments, or where glare situations are constantly present.

During night flight, scotopic rod vision is needed to see other aircraft, and for landing. Complete dark adaptation for good peripheral vision takes about thirty minutes, so a pilot must be careful not to subject himself to bright light while flying at night, unless completely unavoidable. Peripheral or "off-center" viewing is important while flying at night since fixating on a faintly lit object picked up in the peripheral visual field will cause the pilot to lose sight of it. The reason for this is that the foveal cones are much less sensitive to light than the peripheral rods. Red cockpit lighting, permitting photopic cone vision inside the cockpit, is used to preserve scotopic vision for viewing outside the cockpit. It is this frequency of light to which the rods are least sensitive.

There are several visual illusions to which pilots can be subjected while flying. Many of these can be avoided or overcome through conditioning, and by certain viewing techniques. Autokinesis, where a fixed light is seen to move when stared at, can occur in daylight when staring at an object against a uniform background. This situation is more usual at night when a pilot stares at a fixed, lit object against a black background. This visual illusion causes spatial disorientation and probably accounts for some of the accidents which occur during night landings. The physiologic basis for this illusion is felt to be an increase in ocular microsaccades due to poor peripheral visual fixation cues. Its appearance is facilitated by darkness, the presence of only a single light of low intensity, prolonged fixation of gaze, and fatigue. This should not be any problem for the pilot who maintains the aforementioned scanning procedure, where fixations are no more than a few seconds.

Another visual illusion to which pilots can be subjected is the oculogravic or vestibulovisual illusion. A pilot will notice apparent motion of a visual reference point (or portions of it) while he is being subjected to definite changes in acceleration, such as when the force of gravity decreases or disappears. Immobile objects will acquire an illusory movement in the direction of the resultant accelerative force. It is felt that this illusion results from a central integration of the feedback signals from the oculomotor muscles. These muscles are subjected to vestibular tonic influences from the simultaneous stimulation of the otolithic apparatus and semicircular canals, when the acceleration changes. The practical significance of this illusion is moot. It is probably only important that the pilot, who performs flight maneuvers where he might be subjected to forces which bring on this illusion, be aware that his visual perception may not be a totally accurate picture of his surroundings for those few seconds while he is performing the maneuver.

A visual illusion less likely to be a problem for pilots in earth-bound aircraft is the oculogyric illusion. It is observed as an apparent movement of objects in the field of vision, or in the field of vision movement itself, when the individual is subjected to angular accelerations stimulating the vestibular apparatus. The psychophysiologic basis for this illusion is unclear.

PILOT REACTION TO ACCELERATIVE FORCES AND HIGH ALTITUDES

A pilot performing aerobatics or certain maneuvers, such as pulling out of a dive or making a steep banking turn, can be subjected to forces (acceleration or deceleration) which can severely affect his visual and physical performance in flying his aircraft. In general, both physical and physiological factors determine man's resistance to acceleration effects. Individual resistance, dependent on health, age, training, psychologic preparation and motivation, is the most important physiologic factor. The physical factors affecting pilot performance are the magnitude of acceleration, duration of application, position of the pilot's body and extremities with respect to the accelerative force vectors, acceleration rise gradient, and the use of protective systems and body restraints. Environmental conditions such as temperature and pressure also affect pilot performance.

APPENDIX II

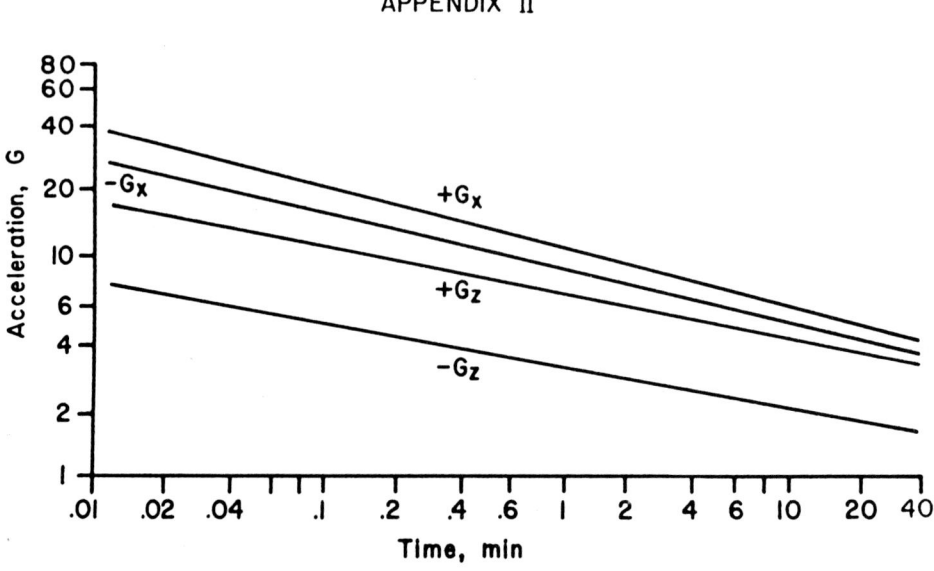

Figure 8-1. Man's resistance to the effects of acceleration in various directions. Mean data on $+G_z$ (head to pelvis), $-G_z$ (pelvis to head), $+G_x$ (chest to back), $-G_x$ (back to chest) (direction of inertial forces).

Man is least resistant to accelerative forces directed along the axis from pelvis to head and most resistant to accelerative forces directed from chest to back. The G-suit is a specially designed garment which constricts the lower parts of the body and prevents the pooling of blood. A pilot not wearing this suit when encountering accelerative forces in the head to foot direction of 4.5 to 6.0 times the force of gravity for more than six seconds, can expect to lose his peripheral vision (grey-out) and then his central vision (black-out), just before losing consciousness. This is probably due primarily to insufficiency in the retinal circulation, although vascular insufficiency in the posterior visual pathways is undoubtedly a concomitant occurrence. Low levels of accelerative forces can cause decreases in visual acuity and increases in reaction times prior to the onset of grey-out. Several seconds (8 to 10) after the application of a constant accelerative force of several G, the pilot will sometimes recover normal vision and reaction times as the homeostatic cardiovascular reflexes compensate for the hemodynamic changes. (Fig. 8-1)

Man is least tolerant of accelerative forces from the foot to head, where the limit is only 2.5 to 3 times the force of gravity for several seconds. This causes "red-out" which results from venous and capillary congestion in the retina. Transverse forces on the body are well tolerated up to 20 G for several seconds, and do not impair visual function to the extent of other body systems. For example, the sitting reclined position of the astronauts in their rockets at lift-off produces forces of only 6 to 8 G.

Visual function can be adversely affected by hypoxia in high altitude flying in addition to the accelerative forces just mentioned. Normally, oxygen use is required by the Federal Aviation Regulations (FAR 91.32) for pilots flying in excess of thirty minutes above an altitude of 12,500 feet or 3810 m. Oxygen is required as back-up for crew and passengers in pressurized aircraft, in case of decompression, at any altitudes flown over 14,000 feet or 4270 m. If, by some accident, a pilot is subjected to hypoxia at high altitudes, visual function suffers commensurate with mental and other bodily functions. Above 43,000 feet (13,100 m), unconsciousness can occur within fifteen seconds. Death can occur within minutes. Above 35,000 feet (9140 m), unconsciousness occurs within one minute and above 23,000 feet (7010 m), in several minutes. Above 12,000 feet (3810 m), although consciousness may not be lost, the pilot suffers from impairment of judgment and visual function, poor fine motor coordination, drowsiness, and light-headedness.

Ophthalmic findings occasionally seen within several hours when individuals ascend to high altitudes are confined to the retinal vasculature and include arterial and venous dilatation, vascular tortuosity, intraretinal hemorrhages, optic disc hyperemia, and an increased retinal blood flow. The incidence and severity of these findings have been noted to increase as the altitude increases. There have been no reports of these findings in pilots who use oxygen at altitudes above 12,500 feet, and are generally in a pressurized aircraft. The greater exertional level of a mountain climber may predispose him to a higher incidence of retinal hemorrhages than a pilot flying at the same altitude. Clearly, pilots are subjected to hypoxic environments less frequently and for shorter periods of time as a result of legal requirements, and therefore, they are less apt to manifest the retinal changes discussed above.

Other factors that cause poor pilot performance also affect visual performance to some extent. These factors include smoking, toxic gas accumulation (carbon monoxide), fatigue, general health, and many medications. Obviously, any of these factors which can affect the mental or visual status of the pilot may be a serious and life-threatening problem during the performance of critical aircraft maneuvers.

Eye injuries (and injuries in general) as a result of the activity of flying (as opposed to crashing) are probably very rare. Retinal damage from overexposure to light, such as glare, is conceivable at high altitudes where less of the sun's ultraviolet rays are filtered, due to the thinner atmosphere. When performing an aerobatic maneuver known as an outside loop, where the accelerative force is directed from pelvis to head, it is possible for a pilot to suffer from retinal hemorrhages (possibly depending on his intraocular pressure). When flying in an open air cockpit or balloon without protective goggles, ocular foreign bodies are a common occurrence. Generally speaking, when a pilot is in a cockpit, he is in a closed environment which lends itself to safety provided he can maintain some sort of equilibrium, with the outside environment. If he cannot, then his visual function will probably be the least of his troubles!

APPENDIX I

Visual Requirements for First-Class Medical Certificate (Federal Aviation Regulations, Part 67.13(b).)

1. Distant visual acuity of 20/20 or better in each eye separately, without correction; or of at least 20/100 in each eye separately corrected to 20/20 or better with corrective lenses (glasses or contact lenses) in which case the applicant may be qualified only on the condition that he wears those corrective lenses while exercising the privileges of his airman certificate.
2. Near vision of at least $v = 1.00$ at 18 inches with each eye separately, with or without corrective glasses.
3. Normal color vision.
4. Normal fields of vision.
5. No acute or chronic pathological condition of either eye or adenexae that might interfere with its proper function, might progress to that degree, or might be aggravated by flying.
6. Bifoveal fixation and vergencephoria relationships sufficient to prevent a break in fusion under conditions that may reasonably occur in performing airman duties.

Tests for the factors named in subparagraph (6) of this paragraph are not required except for applicants found to have more than one prism diopter of hyperphoria, six prism diopters of esophoria or six prism diopters of exophoria. If these values are exceeded, the Federal Air Surgeon may require the applicant to be examined by a qualified eye specialist to determine if there is bifoveal fixation and adequate vergencephoria relationship. However, if the applicant is otherwise qualified, he is entitled to a medical certificate pending the results of the examination.

Visual Requirements for Second-Class Medical Certificate (Federal Aviation Regulations, Part 67.15(b).)

1. Distant visual acuity of 20/20 or better in each eye separately, without correction; or of at least 20/100 in each eye separately corrected to 20/20 or better with corrective lenses (glasses or contact lenses) in which case the applicant may be qualified only on the condition that he wears those corrective lenses while exercising the privileges of his airman certificate.

2. Enough accommodation to pass a test prescribed by the Administrator based primarily on ability to read official aeronautical maps.
3. Normal fields of vision.
4. No pathology of the eye.
5. Ability to distinguish aviation signal red, aviation signal green, and white.
6. Bifoveal fixation and vergencephoria relationship sufficient to prevent a break in fusion under conditions that may reasonably occur in performing airman duties.

Tests for the factors named in subparagraph (6) of this paragraph are not required except for applicants found to have more than one prism diopter of hyperphoria, six prism diopters of esophoria, or six prism diopters of exophoria. If these values are exceeded, the Federal Air Surgeon may require the applicant to be examined by a qualified eye specialist to determine if there is bifoveal fixation and adequate vergencephoria relationship. However, if the applicant is otherwise qualified, he is entitled to a medical certificate pending the results of the examination.

Visual Requirements for Third-Class Medical Certificate (Aviation Regulations, Part 67.17(b).)

1. Distant visual acuity of 20/50 or better in each eye separately, without correction; or if the vision in either or both eyes is poorer than 20/50 and is corrected to 20/30 or better in each eye with corrective lenses (glasses or contact lenses), the applicant may be qualified on the condition that he wears those corrective lenses while exercising the privileges of his airman certificate.
2. No serious pathology of the eye.
3. Ability to distinguish aviation signal red, aviation signal green, and white.

BIBLIOGRAPHY

1. Federal Aviation Regulations, Part 67, Medical Standards and Certification. Available from the Dept. of Transportation — Federal Aviation Administration, Washington, D.C.
2. *The New Encyclopedia Britannica.* 15th edition, Macropedia Vol. 1: 123-129, 142-147.
3. Berens, C., and Sheppard, B. (Eds.): *Abstracts on Military and Aviation Ophthalmology and Visual Sciences,* Washington, D.C., Biological Sciences Foundation, Ltd.
4. *Medical Handbook for Pilots.* Aviation Circular 67-2, U.S. Dept. of Transportation, Federal Aviation Administration, Washington, D.C., Gov. Printing Office.
5. Moses, Robert A., (Ed): *Adler's Physiology of the Eye: Clinical Applications.* St. Louis, Mosby, 1981.
6. Lubin, J.R., Renne, D., Hackett, D., and Albert, D.M.: High altitude retinal hemorrhage: a clinical and pathological case report. *Ann of Ophthalmol, 14:* 1071, 1982.
7. Mohler, S.R.: *Medication and Flying: A Pilot's Guide.* Boston, Flying, 1982.
8. Whiteside, T.C.D.: *The Problems of Vision in Flight at High Altitude.* London, Butterworth, 1957.
9. Calvin, M. and Gazenko, O.G., (Eds.): *Foundations of Space Biology and Medicine.* Washington, D.C., NASA, 1975, vol. II., 1975.
10. Heath, Donald and Williams, David R.: *Man at High Altitude: The Pathophysiology of Acclimatization and Adaption.* 2nd ed., Churchill-Livingstone, p. 307, 1981.

CHAPTER 9

BASEBALL OPHTHALMOLOGY

FRANK B. HOEFLE

INTRODUCTION

ALTHOUGH the average eye care practice will have very few, if any, professional baseball players, it will certainly have many little leaguers, some with a potential future in baseball. Hopefully, some of the information that follows will help put these youngsters in a position to do their best. There are some very characteristic aspects to the examination, visual correction and treatment of injuries if one is dealing with a patient who is a ball player. One can even suggest to a young player what position on the field he is visually best suited for. If a player is locked into a position, the form of correction of ammetropia may depend on what that position is.

VISUAL DEMANDS IN BASEBALL

Fielding

The visual demands in baseball vary widely according to the position played. Generally, the visual demands in baseball are very high, as in hockey or squash; the demand being a function of the size of the ball, its speed and its distance from the player. A major league pitch can come in at ninety mph and do so in about 0.5 seconds. A line drive can go back out at the same speed.

Pitchers

Pitchers probably have the least visual demand of any fielder, and players with myopia, astigmatism, or any visual problem tend to gravitate to pitching. Major league pitchers are often big, strong youngsters with good arms who are poor outfielders and hitters, many times because of a less than maximum degree of vision.

There are many major league pitchers who wear contact lenses, two on the 1984 New York Mets alone. A few wear glasses, but we feel that contacts are safer, as even safety glasses can become missiles if hit with a line drive. Aside from a return line drive (catching it is usually a matter of luck even with 20/10 vision), the biggest demand on a pitcher is seeing the catcher's signal. This can be a definite problem for a minor league or college player playing night games in their traditionally dim ball parks. For this reason, all Mets minor leaguers have an annual refraction, and pitchers' glasses and contacts are kept current. We try to get as many pitchers as possible into contacts for two reasons, other than safety. When a ball is thrown hard, glasses will often fly off, and glasses tend to steam up when the player perspires.

Catchers

Next to pitchers, catchers tend to be the players with the least visual demand. A 20/20 letter subtends an arc of five minutes with respect to the retina. A baseball is about three inches in diameter, and when thrown from sixty feet, provides an image of almost fifteen minutes of arc when it leaves the pitcher's hand, i.e., a person with 20/40 vision would see the ball, although it might look fuzzy.

The catcher's biggest visual demand would be hitting, as he is expected to do that with some ability. The figures above apply to hitting as well as to catching, except that in catching, the catcher knows where the ball is going. There are several major league catchers who wear glasses or contact lenses. With a mask in place, glasses seem perfectly safe.

Infielders

As a rule, infielders have good vision. If they do not, they tend to gravitate toward pitching or catching, or just drop out of baseball after little league. At ninety feet or so, one can see the ball easily with 20/25 vision, so the acuity demand is not as severe as in the outfield, but the ball, if hit squarely, is traveling quickly and good reaction is necessary. The soft contact lens has been a boon to infielders as dust was a true enemy of the hard lens. More infielders are wearing contacts each year.

Outfielders

The outfielder is the man with the most severe visual demands, perhaps more severe than in any other sport. Aside from being expected to bat with power and for average, he must see a ball in the outfield as soon as possible after it is hit, in order to get his "jump" on the ball. This is particularly true in center field, and even more so if the player is not blessed with exceptional speed and agility.

If a center fielder is three hundred feet from home plate, a three inch baseball subtends an arc of less than five minutes (the height of the 20/20 letter). Five minutes of arc at three hundred feet is 5.2 inches. Therefore, a potential or actual center fielder should have at least 20/15 vision. Stereopsis, as a factor in total visual ability, is also maximally required of outfielders because it plays a role in telling them where to go to intersect the flight of the ball when it reaches six feet above the ground.

Physicists have long been interested in the ability of a man to field a fly ball. In 1968, Seville Chapman of Cornell Aeronautics Laboratory suggested a trigonometric theory.[1] This theory depended solely upon the fielder's visual assessment of the rate of increase or decrease of the tangent of the angle of elevation of the ball. Later workers found this theory untenable as it did not take into account the effect of aerodynamic drag on the ball. They concluded that head movement played a role and this implicated the middle ear in the equation. I believe that the explanation for fielding ability is simply that it is a talent acquired through trial and error (experience). One has only to watch inexperienced little league outfielders to know that the outfielders' ability is not inborn. Interestingly, little leaguers will almost universally come in on a ball hit to them, or hit over their heads. It is no secret that the most frequently misjudged ball, even in the majors, is the ball hit directly at you. In theory, your only clues are the size and height of the ball; you do not see the arc. If a fly ball is hit to one side or the other, you can see the aerodynamic arc progress, and having learned this arc, anticipate the landing zone. Major leaguers frequently circle under a ball that is hit directly at them.

In any event, it is the eye practitioner's responsibility to be sure his center fielders have good vision and good stereopsis. If this is unobtainable, there is an implied responsibility to suggest a transfer of the player to the pitcher's mound.

Hitting

The visual acuity demand in hitting is less than it is in center field. A baseball is three inches in diameter and at sixty feet five minutes of arc, or the size of a 20/20 letter, is only 1.05 inches. In theory, a person with 20/60 vision could see an object the size of a baseball at sixty feet (the 20/60 letter at sixty feet is about three inches tall). But there are additional factors and they are the speed of the ball and its trajectory; for example, the curve, the slider, and the sinker. Since the advent of the center field television camera and slow motion replay, no one doubts that curve balls really do curve and sliders do slide. Bahill, using a computerized system to measure eye movements and a ninety-three mph target ball, has calculated that a player cannot voluntarily visually follow a fastball all the way to the plate.[2] He states that in the last five to ten feet, the ball is going too fast with respect to the observer's eye, and a voluntary saccade is necessary. He further suggests that at some point, one must take an eye off the ball, move over the field of vision ahead of the ball, and pick it up as it enters the new field. He concludes that the batter, through it all, employs saccadic movements, vestibulo-ocular movements, smooth pursuit movements, and vergences.

In any event, there is no doubt that batting is a complex task. My own feeling, at least at the major league level, is that a batter must first be "looking for" a pitch, in other words, guessing whether a fast pitch or a slow one is coming. He actually starts his swing before the ball is thrown (striding in) and then, in the first half of the half second duration of the pitch, he must see the ball, decide if he guessed right, and either stop the swing or go through with it. Since there is so little time for uncertainty, 20/20 acuity to start with is obviously better than 20/60. However, it must be considered that for a hitter, 20/25 with no glasses may be more useful than 20/15 through glasses. Glasses create reflections and perhaps not so occasional smudges. In general, if a professional player has 20/25 or better, we would only prescribe glasses for the outfield. If the vision is 20/30 or worse, we give glasses, and let the player decide on their use. Most players will only accept glasses if the vision is 20/50 or worse, but I have seen several 20/30's with marginal careers, albeit in the majors, that I am sure would have had better "stats" if they had accepted correction.

THE NEW YORK METS EYE EXAM

Professional teams are aware of the importance of vision. Before a player is signed to a professional contract, a scout measures acuity and stereopsis with a battery operated vision tester.

When the newly signed player reports to spring training he is given a complete physical and complete eye examination. These will be repeated yearly while he is with the organization, major league or minor league.

A local eye practitioner is "on call" in each of the hometowns for problems that develop during the year. This is particularly important for players wearing contacts or spectacles, as their schedule and activity does not leave much room for lost and damaged lenses which must be quickly replaced.

In dealing with professional players, one must be thorough in the examination. In addition to the desire to do the best for the patient, his career and the team, there is a very great liability in any undiagnosed health problem that might upset a million dollar a year career. A very significant suit has been generated by the unfortunate stroke suffered by J. Rodney Richards, the Houston Astros pitcher.

The Mets' eye exams are done during spring training in St. Petersburg, Florida, as all of the players, major and minor league, are in the same area at this time. The eye examination consists of the following:

1. History—Many players will not admit that they wear contacts.
2. Visual acuity on a ten foot chart set at twenty feet; acuity measured to 20/10 if possible.
3. Ocular exam and IOP.
4. Confrontation fields (how many fingers).
5. Refraction if necessary.
6. Versions and vergences—red glass or Maddox rod if necessary.
7. Fundus exam.
8. Color vision.
9. Wirt test for stereopsis.
10. Ocular dominance.
11. Anything else necessary.

Each year, over 250 eye exams are performed at the Mets spring training facility in St. Petersburg. The most important exams are, of course, those on the rookies. They are about to have their talents unusually tested in a short period of time, and need every advantage available to be successful. If a player has a refractive error, the time to correct it is at this first examination. The alternative is a lost career (detrimental to the player and to the management) or a career which does not reach full potential. As the years go by, a player who makes the majors is older and less likely to accept correction. One older player refused glasses because he would rather swing at the familiar fuzzy ball rather than at the clear but smaller ball seen through corrective lenses. I am sure there are many in the majors now (I personally know of at least three) who are surviving their mediocre careers when they could be much better players if they would accept correction.

The most important parts of the Mets eye exam are the visual acuity tests and the refraction tests. Vergences can be very important too. One prospective third baseman with a tremendous ability for snaring ground balls, made several errors on pop-ups. He turned out to have a V exotropia and diplopia in upgaze. He was mysteriously traded.

Color vision has not proven to be a problem. We have found several color blind players who did well in the majors. We have also tested ocular dominance to see its effect on batting ability. For many years people have believed that crossed dominance favors a hitter. The theory is that a left-handed hitter has an advantage if his right eye is dominant, as the right eye is the one which sees the pitcher best. We could not disprove this or support it, as the number of crossed dominant players is about the same at every professional level, and the same as the general population. There are a few players in the majors who are naturally right-handed but were taught by their fathers to bat left because the fathers believed in the theory.

CORRECTION OF AMMETROPIA

Spectacles

The following is a description of the spectacles issued to Mets players by our optician, Mr. Bonifide:

1. Plastic lenses are used. The lens material is CR39, such as A.O. Permalite® or Polycarbonate lenses, which are highly scratch resistant. In actual tests, lens surfaces were rubbed with a piece of steel wool to demonstrate the scratch resistant properties. Impact resistance is also necessary.
2. In grinding the lenses, the optical centers are most important as prismatic imbalance must be avoided. There are times when a prism must be ground into a lens in order to accommodate a small Pupillary Distance (P.D.). Most ball players are fitted with frames that are large in area. Such frames have a P.D. much greater than the player's P.D. Therefore, decentration by mechanical means is not possible. The decentration must be accomplished by grinding the prism.

3. Base curves of lenses are important, again to minimize distortions as the player swings his eyes from one edge of the lens to the other. Lenses are usually tinted in very light colors; greys are used and, at times, light beige, to take into consideration the lighting conditions of the ball parks.
4. The frame is fitted as close to the face as is possible, almost form fitted, in order to minimize distortion.
5. Metal frames are used as they are highly resistant to perspiration. The temples are a comfort cable type. A pilot shape is usually preferred, and many times, a head band is used to insure the holding of the frame. Nose bridges of either plastic material or regular nose pad type are offered to the player except in cases where one or the other is noted to accomplish a better fit.
6. A proper pantoscopic tilt is important in order to minimize the apparent rise of the ground.

To summarize, the main factors are proper decentration, base curve, frame size, and proper temple length. The end result will be a pair of spectacles well made and custom fitted.

Contact Lenses

Many professional players, especially catchers, formerly wore hard lenses, but with the advent of the soft lens, many have switched. Hard lenses are difficult in the dust of the infield, and most infielders wear soft lenses or glasses. An outfielder may prefer a hard lens as the quality of vision provided in that visually demanding position is somewhat better. With the newer gas permeable hard lenses, a larger lens can be used to avoid having the player's vision disturbed by seeing the edges. Years ago, some players had small diameter PMMA lenses for general use, and a larger diameter pair for use only during a game. Some had to clear the corneal edema between innings in extra inning games.

Serious baseball players who wear contacts should probably have an eye care professional with them at all times. Their vision is crucial to their performance, but their ability to acknowledge their dependence on their lenses is traditionally pitiful. They almost never have spares, and what they do have is frequently not in top shape. It would be expected that a man who depends on contact lenses to help him earn his $800,000.00 a year, would have six spare pairs; unfortunately, this is often not so.

Baseball players should replace their soft lenses more frequently than the general population. These lenses often become coated, creating a subtle gradual decrease in the quality of vision which a player may not notice, while his batting average is evaporating.

BASEBALL EYE INJURIES AND MEDICAL PROBLEMS

Vinger shows that baseball does account for a large number of sports-related eye injuries.[3] He states that in a series of 159 sports eye injuries from 1977 to 1980, 10 percent were related to baseball. He also states that in another series, 62 percent of the injuries were from the ball, 16 percent from the bat, and 22 percent "unspecified." In a third series of eye injuries, he shows that the greatest number of mishaps is in the five to fourteen year old age group, the little leaguer. This is not surprising as there are certainly more little league players than there are professionals, and a face protector is now available for use in youth baseball.[4] Fortunately, in my eight years with a major league team I have seen only one serious eye injury.

The most common problems that are seen in baseball are:

1. *Actinic conjunctivitis.* There is a phenomenon which I like to call "Shortstops' Eyes" which is probably partly chronic actinic conjunctivitis and partly chronic blepharitis. This condition causes eye rubbing. Whether it is due to the sun, or the dust, or both is moot; nevertheless, many older infielders develop chronic conjunctival injection during the playing season. In general, this condition can easily be controlled with mild medications, but if the tearing and irritation are significant, performance can be affected.
2. *Infectious conjunctivitis.* In any team situation where a group of people are close and often use the nearest towel, the spector of a team infection exists. The trainers in the major leagues are particularly alert to isolating and treating anyone with a painless red eye. The thought of an epidemic in a pennant race is quite frightening.
3. *Contusion of the globe and orbit.* The classic serious baseball eye injury is the contusion of the globe and orbit from a thrown or batted ball. Any or all of the following may occur:

    Hyphema
    Traumatic mydriasis

Dislocated lens
Vitreous hemorrhage
Macular hemorrhage or Berlin's edema
Fractured floor of the orbit

The globe does not rupture because of the size of the ball with respect to the dimensions of the orbit. Fortunately, the full blown injury is rare, but two players (Conigliaro and Score) have had their careers ended.

4. *Tension symptoms.* In assessing a player's eye complaints, it is important to have some knowledge of the player's current performance. A batter in a slump will always blame his eyes. A pitcher who is not doing well will say he cannot see the signs. A few years ago, one player turned up with lid twitching of monumental dimensions. It turned out that he was a nonstarting outfielder-second baseman who was trying to win a starting job at third base. The line drives come very quickly at third. He did not get the job, and the twitching stopped the very next day.

Conclusion

The eyecare professional can have an important role in baseball, whether on the major league level, or on the town team. My association has been a true pleasure. They do not put ophthalmologists in the Hall of Fame, but it is nice to have a couple of patients who are there!

REFERENCES

1. Brancazio, Peter: Physics of judging a fly ball. *Phys Today, 37:* S-5, 1984.
2. Bahill, A. Terry and LaRitz, Tom: Why can't batters keep their eyes on the ball? *Am Sci, 72:* 249, 1984.
3. Vinger, Paul F.: Ocular sports injuries. Principles of protection. *Int. Ophthalmol Clin, 21:* 149, 1981.
4. Tauber, Gil.: Batter up! With eye guards! *Sightsaving, 52:* 10, 1984.

CHAPTER 10

GOLF OPHTHALMOLOGY

CALVIN ROBERTS

"KEEP YOUR HEAD down and watch the ball," is the common plea of a golf instructor. The implication is that the eyes and good vision are helpful for a proper golf swing.

20/20 vision is not, however, necessary to play golf. Tom Watson cannot pass a driving test without glasses, neither can Arnold Palmer. Until recently, Palmer played without spectacles, and Watson still has resisted wearing his myopic correction on the golf course. They are among a large group of people who would not dare drive a car without glasses on but always play golf without correction. Other players, both amateur and professional, find that they play better with glasses than with contact lenses. Still others find that they can wear hard lenses but not soft lenses because the ball looks different.

The role of eyes and, therefore, vision in golf is to provide visual clues for planning the golf swing. If the ball is on a mound, elevated higher than the feet, the player must shorten up or grip the club further down the shaft to create a smaller arc. If the ball is in a gulley, then the golfer must lengthen the arc or lean over toward the ball to compensate.

The brain determines the location of the ball by its spatial relationship to objects such as blades of grass or a golf tee, but more importantly by the apparent size of the ball. If the ball sits farther away it looks smaller or, conversely, it appears larger if it rests closer. An experienced golfer unconsciously uses this information and compensates for the distance of the ball from the body with his swing.

Two examples point out how the eyes can play tricks on a golfer. The "British"-sized golf ball is 1.62 inches in diameter while the "American"-sized golf ball is 1.68 inches in diameter. Though the difference is small, it is readily apparent when the two balls are side by side and even more so when trying to hit the smaller ball for the first time. The brain interprets the smaller size of the ball to mean that it must be farther away, and the golfer tends to lean toward the ball causing the club head to hit the ground first instead of the ball.

A second example is when a player tries to hit a ball that is within a water hazard. Just as a spoon in a glass of water is magnified so is a golf ball in a lake. The larger appearance of the ball causes the golfer to swing over the ball and miss it.

These visual tricks keep golfers from wearing their required optical correction on the golf course. Myopic glasses minify objects while hyperopic glasses magnify. Thus, playing golf with glasses on requires the brain to incorporate this apparent size disparity into its program for determining the position of the golf ball. Many find this adjustment just too difficult. Players who only wear glasses part time leave them off while playing golf and those who wear their glasses full time and whose brain has made the adjustment keep them on.

Contact lenses, positioned closer to the eyes than spectacles, give much less magnification. They are an alternative for the part-time glasses wearer but a disaster to the full-time glasses wearer who has already compensated for the magnification effect of his glasses.

A second key ingredient in planning the golf swing is the knowledge of the distance from the ball to the target. Using the same size/distance type computation, the brain uses the apparent size of the flagstick as an indication of the distance to the hole. Consequently, golf flagsticks are a standard height of 7 1/2 feet to help a golfer assess distances as he plays different golf courses.

To see the size of a flagstick that is 200 yards away does require good acuity. Most golf courses are marked at known distances, therefore professionals carry charts with the distances measured. Still, a common sight is that of Tom Watson squinting at the hole, trying to use his eyelids as pinholes to achieve a better view of the target.

In summary, prior to the swing, the eyes help locate the ball in relation to the stance and help judge the distance to the green and to the hole.

During the swing, ocular pursuits keep the ball on the fovea as the head pivots. The classical description of the pursuit system involves the tracking by the eyes of a moving object while the head stays still. In golf, the object (the ball), is stationary while the head moves. The net result, however, is the same as the eyes rotate to the left during the backswing and back to the right on the downswing.*

Up to this point, the relative acuities of the two eyes have not been of importance for both eyes are open and the ball and target are seen binocularly. However, in the backswing, the right eye's view of the ball becomes obstructed by the nose. Assuming the acuities of the two eyes are the same, the left eye takes over unconsciously. If there is not good vision in the left eye, the brain compensates by restricting the degree of head turn to hold fixation by the right eye. The less the head turns, the more difficult it is to achieve a full shoulder turn on the backswing. The net result is a loss of power on the swing.

On the downswing, the head turns back toward the ball and binocularity is reestablished. At no point is the right eye alone viewing the ball. Thus, a right-handed golfer benefits from good vision in his left eye.

After the ball has been hit, the head turns toward the target so that the eye can follow the flight of the ball. The image of the ball appears first on the peripheral retina and then the saccadic system moves the eyes in order to place this image on the fovea. Once the ball is seen, then the pursuit system allows the eyes to follow the ball to its destination. Golfers with aphakic spectacles find following the ball to be difficult since their peripheral vision is restricted. Also, the jack-in-the-box effect may allow the ball to come in and then out of view before the saccades have had a chance to properly point the eyes at the ball.

No part of the game of golf is dependent on the eyes as much as putting. Not only must a golfer judge the direction to putt the ball and the pace with which it must be hit, but he must orient the blade of the putter accordingly.

To see the line, most golfers squat or bend over so that their eyes are closer to the ground and can better visualize the subtleties of the green's contour. Getting closer to the ground also allows the eyes' parallax system to make fine discriminations on the basis of the slightly different images to the two eyes. Just as binocularity is necessary for depth perception, good vision from both eyes reveals more about the break of the green than does monocularity.

---

*All discussions are in the context of a right-handed swing. For a left-hander, the reverse would be the case.

Sometimes, the parallax view is unsettling, especially when one stands up and the distance from the ground causes the parallax to go to zero, and the green looks different. Therefore, it is not uncommon to see a golfer close one eye when looking from the ground at a putt since it will look more similar to his view of the line when he is ready to putt.

Another means to judge the contour of the green is to hold the shaft of the putter vertically at arms length toward the hole and using one eye only, sight the relative heights of the green at each side of the shaft. Relatively few golfers use this technique, but those who do report that the separation of the two fields makes subtleties easier to judge.

One quality of all good putters is that as they putt, their eyes are aligned directly over the golf ball. Thus, their perception of the envisioned path of the ball corresponds most closely to the view from behind the ball and the roll. Many golfers adopt a putting stance bent at the waist, again, to help their visualization of the break.

Just as the importance of the left eye during the backswing was noted, so does the left eye take on added importance when putting. In preparation to putt, the golfer frequently glances at the hole, then back to the ball, then back to the hole, etc., confirming that his orientation of the putter blade is correct for the desired direction to hit the ball. In a putting stance, with the head facing toward the ball, the nose again partially blocks the view toward the hole. Each time the golfer looks up at the hole, he is using his full visual field. Depending on how much he turns his head to look at the hole, he may be seeing it with the left eye only.

Does this imply that a right-handed golfer whose left eye is dominant has an advantage? Probably so, since at the moments when he is monocular, he is using his dominant eye.

One recent innovation in golf is the use of colored golf balls. Many golfers find that there is less glare when looking at a yellow or pale green ball than with the conventional white ball. Thus, they squint less on a sunny day. Others, particularly those with cataracts or occular degeneration, find the bright orange balls easier to see at a distance against the green backdrop. The primary reason why most golfers have not changed from the white ball is that a different color ball throws off their spatial relationships, similar to that previously discussed when wearing glasses. Any change requires adjustments.

An appreciation of the importance of vision for golf makes it all the more remarkable that the visually handicapped are able to enjoy the game. Using an assistant as their "eyes," these golfers position themselves at the ball, and swing. They use their sense of feel to partially compensate for their lack of vision. Others who have only partial visual impairments learn to compensate for them as they play. This is one reason why golf remains a popular sport even among older people.

REFERENCES

1. Wannebo, M., and Reeve, T.G.: Effects of skill level and sensory information on golf putting. *Percept Mot Skills, 58:* 611, 1984.
2. Akssamit, G., and Husak W.: Feedback influences on the skill of putting. *Percept Mot Skills, 56:* 19, 1983.
3. Getz, D.J.: Vision and sports. *J Am Optom Assoc, 49:* 385, 1978.

CHAPTER 11

THE EYE AND SHOOTING

JAMES A. SALISBURY

THE DESIRE FOR accuracy in shooting provides the impetus for many a marksman to enlist the skills of his eye care professional. There are several optical aids that can be utilized to achieve the consistant precision of marksmanship demanded by modern riflery and shotgunning.

AIMING

Refraction and Basic Principles

Aiming begins with good visual acuity. Wearing lenses of the appropriate refraction produces the clearest retinal image, thereby reducing fatigue and eyestrain. A sportsman aspiring to his expectations must have his best refraction for visual performance. Accurate shooting depends upon the basic principles of vision; fusion, stereopsis, and depth perception.

A wide binocular field of view is important in the initial location of a target. Motion in a peripheral visual field provides the stimulus for the fusion response. This creates a solitary mental image for precise aiming. Without fusion, suppression or diplopia would result. This leads to confusion or the loss of valuable environmental information which is needed in correct target alignment. Good depth perception helps judge not only the target distance but also the relative position of two or more objects in the viewing field.

Uniocular target sighting employs visual clues such as apparent size, perspective, shadows, parallax and overlapping of contours. Muscular clues for depth perception include efforts of accommodation and convergence. Although one may perceive depth by using the above mentioned uniocular clues, binocular stereoscopic vision provides the best means of judging depth. This occurs with the correct interpretation of slightly disparate images.

Correct muscle alignment lessens fatigue and aids the depth perception determination. Castren demonstrated that a heterophoria less than six prism diopters does not affect the stereoscopic vision.[1] Any measurement greater than this leads to early fatigue and/or ocular image suppression.

Eye Dominance

Eye dominance is another important factor in shooting accurately; sighting with the dominant eye is used to align the gun sights with the target. When the nondominant eye aligns the gun and target, the sight image appears good, but the target is missed. This is known as cross firing.

Most sportsmen usually have a strong dominant eye, a factor which contributes to consistant shooting. Others have alternating dominance, occurring with fatigue, stress, or poor lighting conditions. Proper alignment is thus compromised.

Of greater consequence is ocular dominance mismatched with arm dominance. This is less important in such sports as tennis or basketball because one has learned to compensate. With rifle shooting this does not present a problem as one eye is usually closed to align the sights. However, to shoot a shotgun this way, the head must be positioned over the stock or the gun must be twisted to compensate for the nondominant eye alignment.

Many a shooter does not know how to determine which eye is dominant. One way to do this is to focus on a distant object through a small hole cut in a piece of paper held at arm's length. Advance this paper toward your face, keeping the object in focus the entire time. The paper will thus be brought directly to the dominant eye. Another way is to focus on a small object fifteen feet away. While still focusing on the object and with both eyes open, block it out with your thumb held at arm's length from your body. In this position, close one eye. If the object appears to remain blocked by your thumb, the open eye is the dominant eye. If the object appears to jump from behind your thumb, the closed eye is the dominant eye.

Veteran shooters, however, find it easy to learn ways to compensate for cross dominance. One technique is to close the eye not aligned with the gun barrel. This helps force dominance onto the other eye, but interrupts binocular vision. Closing this eye just before firing the gun helps preserve binocular vision. Another technique is to mount an occluder alongside the gun barrel to block the off eye's view. Yet another method is to block the off-aligned eye's view of the end of the gun barrel by putting petroleum jelly or some similar substance on the lens used in shooting. Gun stocks can also be made to permit the dominant eye to be aligned with the barrel when the gun is placed upon the opposite shoulder, although this method is by far the most expensive.

USE OF AIDS IN AIMING

Shooting Glasses

Optical aids that may be used for shooting begin with the shooting glasses. Frames should ride high enough on the nose to be clear of the cheek when the face is aligned against the gun stock. A frame with adjustable nose pads will provide an individualized fit. A larger than customary frame will help eliminate glare. Metal frames or a combination of metal and plastic are more durable than plastic alone. Each frame must conform to the individual's facial contours.

Tinted Lenses, Optical Centers, and Contact Lenses

Distracting glare and brightness can be reduced by tinted lenses. Neutral grey tints will absorb 98 percent of the ultraviolet along with the infrared radiation without distorting color perception. Green tints absorb the infrared rays and 99 percent of the ultraviolet radiation, but are less effective in reproducing true colors and blocking bright light. Brown tints absorb similarly to green tinted lenses, but there is greater color distortion due to less visible blue light being transmitted.

Shooting glasses with yellow tint absorb 100 percent of the ultraviolet rays while transmitting the infrared and 83 percent of the visible spectrum. Scattered light of fog and atmospheric haze is decreased because of the blue region of the spectrum. Subjectively, yellow lenses may be beneficial because they increase contrast, but there is no evidence that they improve one's marksmanship. In summary, different tints produce different combinations of positive and negative factors, and therefore the shooter's individual preferences must be taken into account.

Polaroid lenses decrease annoying surface reflections such as those seen over water or concrete. Antireflective coating decreases individual lens glare by using an ultrathin layer of magnesium fluoride.

Alignment of the optical centers of the shooting lenses must be achieved to produce the sharpest vision without inducing any prism effect. Sighting for pistols usually requires looking through the upper right or left corner of a lens. Gun stock shape will determine eye alignment for rifles and shotguns, but sighting is usually through the upper left edge of the lens for the right-hander and the upper right corner for left-handers. Regardless of the sighting position, viewing is usually high in the lens, and the optical centers must be properly aligned.

Contact lenses offer aid to the sportsman by affording good central and peripheral vision. There are no troublesome lens reflections, no frame adjustments and no optical center problems, but contact lenses afford virtually no eye protection. The latter is reason enough to reconsider their value to the marksman unless protective glasses are worn in combination with them.

Open and Aperture Sights

In addition to aids for better vision, there are aids for better aiming. These aiming aids are the open sight and the aperture sight on the gun itself.

Open sights are the iron sights customarily present on a rifle or pistol. They usually consist of a rear notch and a front bead. With vision fully corrected, the downrange target is in focus while the rear sight and front bead are always slightly out of focus. Because of this blurriness, hurried shots commonly result in a vertically misaligned shot, and therein lies the open sight's weakness. Horizontal hold is fairly easy to obtain with the rear notch limiting lateral displacement. Most hunting shots are taken at targets less than 200 yards away. Open sights work fairly well at distances of 150 to 250 yards.

The aperture, or peep sight, is another aiming aid. Wearing the best refraction is required, as with open sights. The aperture creates parallel rays of light that enter the eye. The smaller the aperture, the less light, but the better the optical effect.

The depth of field created by the aperture is dependent upon projection distance and the distance separating the aperture from the eye. An adjustable iris aperture will allow a small aperture for targeting shooting or a larger aperture for aligning moving targets such as game.

One disadvantage of both open and aperture sights is that a portion of the target is blocked. This blockage is not a critical factor for range shooting, but it does hinder game identification while hunting.

Scopes

Telescopic gunsights are still another aid used for aiming. A scope will provide an instant sighting with proper reticle alignment, thus eliminating most problems of shooter eye focus. This is advantageous for the presbyope who has difficulty focusing with the iron sights. Minor corrective errors can be adjusted in the scope's eye piece, but large refractive errors should be corrected with the proper corrective lenses.

Target alignment through a scope depends upon the field of view, the stock design, and exit pupil size. With the most popular American hunting scope powers (2 1/2×, 3×, 4×, and 6×) the field of view becomes a small issue because the new side-angle scopes enable few detectable differences among them.

Stock design is important for quick eye alignment. A stock which easily positions the eye behind the scope usually is one with a high, thick comb; the comb being the area where the cheek touches the stock.

The exit pupil controls the amount of light exiting a scope. This narrow pencil of light enters the central aspect of the pupil, a location more visually efficient than a peripheral entrance (Stiles-Crawford effect), and affects the acuity with which the field of view is perceived.

The size of the exit pupil regulates the amount of light entering the eye. The exit pupil's size is calculated by dividing the millimeter diameter of the objective lens in the scope by the power of the scope. The larger the exit pupil, the easier the eye can pick up the entire field of view.

A large exit pupil entering a large pupil will help with alignment but adds nothing when shooting. For example, in dim light the pupil may be dilated to five millimeters. A scope with an exit pupil larger than five millimeters is not needed. A 4× scope with a thirty-two millimeter objective has an eight millimeter exit pupil. Again, this large zone aids in quick alignment, but adds nothing when shooting with this large pupil. All the light the eye can use is being supplied to it by an exit pupil equivalent in size to the eye's pupil.

Contrary to belief, scopes do not gather light. They lose light depending upon the number of lenses contained within the system and the quality of the lens coating. Visibility at dusk is better through a scope because the target seems closer. Visibility does not continue to improve with higher scope powers. In a 9× scope with a thirty millimeter objective, only a 3.3 millimeter exit pupil enters a five millimeter dilated pupil. The resultant image is low in contrast and produces a "washed out" image.

Focusing a scope first means adjusting the ocular lens. The presbyope or mild hyperope will adjust the ocular lens by turning it outward, while the myope will turn it inward.

The second focus problem is eliminating parallax, the objective lens focus error. One uses the cross hairs as the middle reference plane. If the cross hairs move with the eye movement, the objective lens is set for too short a distance. If they move opposite the eye movement, the objective is set for too great a distance. This movement interferes with depth perception and accuracy. Gross parallax error can be eliminated by establishing a stabilized head position and aligning the eye through the center of the scope.

High-powered scopes increase resolution and aid in interpreting image drift. A mirage is created by light being refracted in varying degrees through a layered temperature gradient. Some of the image displacement that results can be compensated for by using the higher-powered scopes.

A mirage effect is also created from a hot gun barrel. This mirage is unrelated to the ground mirage of the actual shooting condition. Tubular scope extensions used mainly by bench competition marksmen eliminate the barrel mirage.

One other point that should be mentioned when discussing scopes is their mounting. Scopes must be mounted at the proper distance from the eye in order to avoid the painful experience of being struck over the eyebrow by a heavy magnum. This distance should be at least three and one-half inches, and most good scopes allow for at least three-quarters of an inch further latitude of eye relief.

SHOTGUN, RIFLE, AND PISTOL AIMING

Different weapons require different sighting techniques; those needed for shotgun sighting may vary considerably from those necessary in rifle or pistol shooting.

Aiming a shotgun effectively requires that both eyes be open, with the dominant eye down against the gun stock in line with the barrel. Accuracy depends upon target concentration rather than on the weapon. The idea is to shoot where you look, rather than to take specific aim. The proficient shotgunner has mastered this technique.

The target games of trap and skeet, in which the shotgun is used, create some optical illusion. In trap shooting, the target appears to be going horizontally straight away from the shooter, but in fact, it is rising quite rapidly. A higher special stock or bent-up barrel will help compensate for this illusion.

In skeet shooting it appears that the target is not traveling as fast as the required lead or forward allowance necessary to hit it. The speed of the target in American skeet is roughly fifty miles per hour. Another illusion created in skeet shooting is the target distance, especially from stations three, four, and five. (There are eight shooting stations. Stations one through seven, numbered from left to right, are spaced equally throughout a 180 degree arc, with station eight being the center of the arc's circle.) The distance appears to be thirty yards, but to the center of the crossing point it is actually only twenty-one yards. Once the tricks are learned in both trap and skeet shooting, the percentage of hit targets will most certainly increase.

Sighting of a rifle usually is done with the nonaiming eye or "off eye" closed or suppressed. The iron sights of a rifle are aligned and centered on the target. Focus is on the target, which creates a slight blur on the edges of the open sights. Because the sights are only used for centering the target, this minor blurring is not of any consequence. Accurate pistol shooting requires precise focusing of the front sight. This creates a slight blur to the downrange target as the sights are aligned and focused on it. Properly refracted lenses should be worn for the necessary clarity.

The presbyope may require a special shooting lens for pistol marksmanship. One of two methods to aid focus is altering the prescription in the shooting glasses to achieve a clear focus on the front sight. Only the shooting eye will need this modification in lens power.

The presbyope's plus power can be added to plain shooting glasses in two ways. A flip-over lens or a flip-up front frame can hold the needed power. Still another way of providing the plus power is to use a tiny bifocal placed in the corner of the glass through which aim is taken. A round fused bifocal usually works well.

Another approach presbyopes utilize is a pinhole on the spectacle lens. The lens is marked with a wax china marking pencil directly in the line of sight. A pinhole approximately 1.5 millimeters in diameter in a 3/8 inch wide strip of black electrician's tape is then placed precisely over the marked spot. Trial and error will indicate the best pinhole size for the amount of illumination. This pinhole will increase the apparent depth or range of clear focus. The single pinhole is usually for a one-hand hold support. If both one and two hands are to be used in the course of a shooting day, a wider piece of tape with a second pinhole placed closer to the center line may be used. Adjustable diaphragms may be purchased to produce this tiny aperture. With a smaller aperture the focus is clearer, but the illumination is reduced.

Tape can also be used to help block the unsuppressed eye in pistol shooting. The dominant eye usually aligns the pistol sights on the target. If closing the nondominant eye creates unnecessary tension, the double image can be blocked with a piece of tape. For the right-handed shooter the tape is placed in the upper right-hand corner of the left lens, and in the upper left corner of the right lens for the left-hander.

Focusing and accommodative amplitude may be affected by several different things. The uncorrected hyperope or a shooter with Adie's Syndrome may present as a premature presbyope. True presbyopic symptoms may be caused by marked hypothyroidism, severe anemia, myasthenia gravis, diabetes, or open angle glaucoma. Drugs taken long and short-term can affect accommodation. Some of the more commonly known drugs to have this side effect are the parasympatholytics, phenothiazines, chloroquine, sulfonamides, tetracyclines, and the carboanhydrase inhibitors. The myope who is prepresbyopic and changes to contact lens wear must now exert more accommodative effort for his near focus.

INJURIES: PREVENTION AND TREATMENT

Eye injuries caused by a BB, pellet, or lead shot usually present in an "all or none" phenomenon with regard to prognosis. Either a glancing blow with minimal trauma is experienced, or severe contussive damage and penetration with deformation of the globe occur. Bowen reported that the two main causes for resultant poor vision from ocular injuries caused by air gun pellets were retinal damage and cataract.[2] Drummond reported that 85 percent of his twenty cases on ocular perforation due to shotgun pellets had a resultant visual acuity of hand motion or worse.[3]

Ocular perforation can occur when the speed of the missile reaches a velocity of approximately forty meters per second.[4] Table 11-1[5,6] compares the muzzle velocities of various powder and nonpowder firearms which discharge pellets. It is easy to see that both the powder and nonpowder firearms easily generate missile velocities capable of perforating the globe.

Table 11-1

MUZZLE VELOCITIES OF FIREARMS WHICH DISCHARGE PELLETS

Type of Firearm	Muzzle Velocity (m/sec)
Spring BB gun rifle	84-99
CO2 gun	145-152
Pump pellet gun:	
2 pumps	117
4 pumps	158
6 pumps	181
8 pumps	194
10 pumps	206
Shotgun	259

Everyone should wear safety glasses when discharging firearms. Debris from discharging powder and tiny particles of brass are hurled toward the eye upon extraction and ejection of the fired cartridge case.

The Food and Drug Administration ruled that all lenses produced after December 31, 1971, must be impact-resistant, except where specified by the eye care provider that visual needs would be impaired.[7] Robertson demonstrated that chemically-tempered lenses afford more protection than plastic or heat-tempered lenses.[8] The new polycarbonate lenses can easily withstand the impact of a BB pellet. Nicks and scratches weaken a lens, so damaged or worn lenses should be replaced. Eye protection is necessary to help avoid injury in an environment where firearms are being discharged; therefore, it is good practice for the observer as well as the participant to wear protective eye gear. Adolescents should be taught that no guns should be considered as toys.

Since ocular trauma from firearms is potentially devastating, both sportsman and spectator alike should be well versed in the rules of gun safety and etiquette. Proper usage and handling of firearms is of utmost importance in the prevention of ocular morbidity.

REFERENCES

1. Castren, J., Rutanen, H., and Aho, J.: On the significance of heterophoria for stereoscopic vision. *Aviat Space Environ Med, 53:* 393, 1982.
2. Bowen, D.I., and Magauran, D.: Ocular injuries caused by airgun pellets. *Br Med J, 1:* 333, 1973.
3. Drummond, J., and Kieler, R.A.: Perforating ocular shotgun injuries. *South Med J, 69:* 1066, 1976.
4. Dimaio, V.J.M.: Penetration of skin by bullets and missles. *Forensic Sci Gazette, 11:* 1, 1980.
5. Product Information. Daisy Division, Victor Comptometer Corp., Rogers, Arkansas.
6. Drye, J.C., and Schuster, G.: Shotgun wounds. *Am J Surg, 85:* 438, 1953.
7. Statements of general policy or interpretation: Use of impact-resistant lenses in eyeglasses and sunglasses. *Federal Register.* Title 21: Food and Drugs. Chapter 1, Subchapter A, Part 3. *37:* 2503, 1972.
8. Robertson, D.M.: Safety glasses as protection against shotgun pellets. *Am J Ophthalmol, 81:* 671, 1976.

FOR FURTHER READING

1. Barsness, John: What is this thing on my rifle and why am I looking through it? *Gray's Sporting J, 4:* 12, 1979.
2. Brister, Bob: *Shotgunning: the Art and Science.* Tulsa, Winchester Press, 1976.
3. Duke-Elder, S.: The physiology of the eye and of vision. *In Systems of Ophthalmology,* St. Louis, Mosby, 1968, Vol. IV.
4. Gregg, James R.: *The Sportsman's Eye.* Tulsa, Winchester Press, 1971.
5. Kojovic, V., and Purisic, S.: Influence of side effects of some drugs upon visual functions and results in sport shooting. *Med Arh, 36:* 201, 1982.
6. MacDaniel, Donald: Pistol shooters RX for tired eyes. *Amer Rifleman, 132:* 1984.
7. Milder, Benjamin, and Rubin, Melvin L.: *The Fine Art of Prescribing Glasses Without Making a Spectacle of Yourself.* Gainesville, Triad Sci Pub., 1978.
8. Page, Warren: *The Accurate Rifle.* South Hackensack, N.J., Stoeger, 1973.

CHAPTER 12

WINTER SPORTS: HOCKEY AND SKIING

Alain P. Rousseau, Marcel Amyot, and Pierre F. Labelle

VISUAL REQUIREMENTS

Hockey and skiing call for astute visual performance when participants attain a certain level of excellence. Yet, both sports are actively practiced by individuals with little or no residual vision. Such "blind" hockey teams exist in Canada, particularly in Quebec and Ontario; they play against teams composed of seeing players. Goaltenders on both sides are usually completely blind, while the other players have some degree of residual vison. The puck is replaced by a tin can painted black; physical contacts are, of course, prohibited (Fig. 12-1).

An international association for blind skiers supports competitions for the completely and legally blind. Many nonseeing also ski for pleasure. Runs are usually chosen so that unexpected surface irregularities are avoided. The blind skier follows or skies close to a seeing leader who signals his position by sound; both usually wear "blind skier" signs fastened to their back and front. Although both sports are accessible to the blind, a better visual status is necessary for higher competitive activities. Varying degrees of visual function are required for different levels of expertise in skiing and hockey.

Skiing and hockey share one characteristic, speed, which requires sharpness in the perception of image, brisk visual reflexes, and an increased awareness of the surroundings for rapid motor response. Good illumination, while usually available in each sport, is subject to variations in skiing, owing to meteorologic conditions. Training will neither

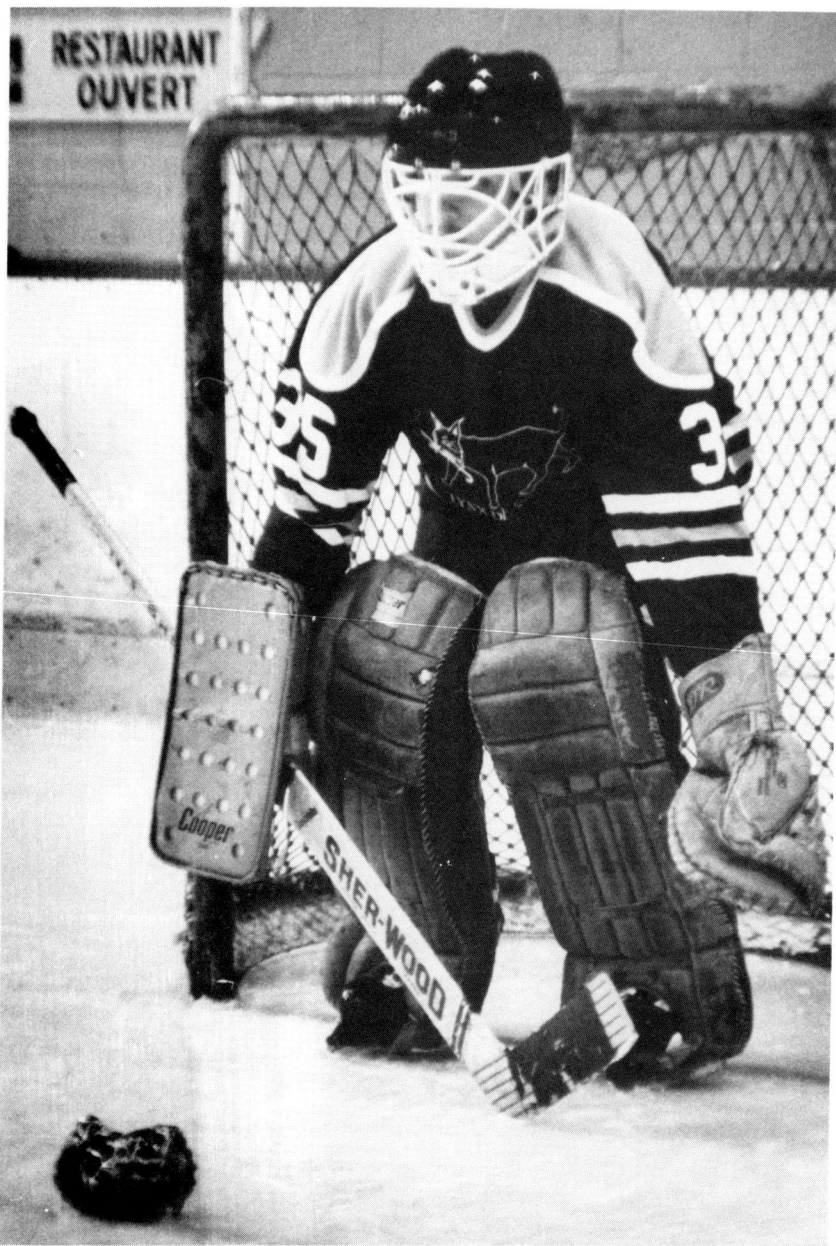

Figure 12-1. Blind hockey players use a tin can instead of the regular hockey puck.

improve visual acuity nor enlarge the visual field. Training can, however, improve overall effectiveness by increasing concentration, and possibly by developing an awareness of peripheral vision for static and moving targets. Evaluation of the speed of a moving object in the peripheral field could also be improved.[1]

Skiing

For pleasure, skiing does not necessarily demand excellent vision, but as one acquires skills and reaches a level closer to competition, visual acuity and adequate visual reflexes are of utmost importance. Curiously, the Canadian National Ski Team has neither visual requirements nor performs an ocular examination prior to enlisting members.

Adequate visual acuity appropriate to the type of skiing practiced is necessary to anticipate surface irregularities, contrasts, contours of moguls, and sudden drops to avoid loss of balance and possible accidents. This is of particular importance in cloudy and snowing conditions, wherein the snow takes a somewhat uniform color thereby obscuring drops. Towards the end of the day, vision is always reduced, secondary to fatigue and lighting alterations.[1,2]

Color vision might not be as crucial as in other sports and color deficits should not pose a severe handicap. Coding of the degrees of difficulty of the slopes are monitored both through colors and shapes of the signs.

The visual field should be comparable to that required for driving a car. One should be aware of oncoming skiers to avoid collisions, particularly where runs converge at the lower part of the mountain. The kinetic field of vision, which enables one to identify a moving target and the speed of the object in the peripheral field, is of increasing importance as the speed of the skier is increased.

Illumination is an imporant factor which, ideally, should be neither too bright as to cause glare nor too dim as to decrease the shades and contours of the moguls. Poor or slow dark adaptation might be an inconvenience to a competitive skier.

Stereopsis requires and is the ultimate reward of binocular vision. It is most important to enable the skier to detect unevenness in the runs, appreciate distance, and anticipate proper movements and position. Stereopsis is particularly necessary in slalom competition and in jumping where one needs to appreciate the doors in slalom and the distance to the jump take-off. Deficits could be partly compensated by monocular clues for the well-trained monocular individual, and would not constitute a major handicap for an ocular defect dating from birth. Deficits would, however, be of considerable disadvantage to a skier who lost an eye through an accident later in life. A longer adaptation would undoubtedly be necessary, and might be unattainable.

There are intrinsic and extrinsic factors to which skiers must adapt. Among intrinsic factors, fatigue, towards the end of the day, decreases both visual performance as well as powers of concentration. Altitude must be accounted for as many ski centers are situated 8,000 to 12,000 feet above sea level and the skier changes altitude rapidly and frequently. A 4,000 feet variation in altitude repeated at rapid rate is significant. This factor requires a few days for adaptation, as hypoxia manifests itself at the beginning, and affects both the brain and the retina.[1,2] A period of adaptation (acclimation) is necessary prior to skiing at high altitudes. Moreover, one would do well to improve one's physical fitness prior to undertaking high altitude skiing. At high altitudes, visual acuity decreases as a result of hypoxia and adaptation to variation in illumination is definitely slower, as confirmed by Wiedman.[3]

Speed is an important facet of skiing and one tends to match progress with greater velocity. Therein lies the "challenge and danger." It must be kept in mind that the latent period between perception, integration of information, and a motor response is close to half a second. As speed increases, adequate knowledge and anticipation of the conditions that will be encountered should compensate for poorer visual perception.

White-out effect, prevalent under foggy conditions, may occur when skiing off-trail, particularly above tree lines. When fully expressed, the skier looses all visual references, contours disappear, and the slopes, moguls, and pits flatten. Vision decreases secondary to a loss of accommodation and points of reference. A sensation of the ground moving under one's feet and vertigo are experienced, anxiety develops, and the skier feels a need to rest on his poles. At this point, it is impossible to distinguish a hill from a precipice, hence, conditions are prime for serious accidents.

Should competition be made available to the one-eyed skier? If the loss of vision dates from birth, the athlete has compensated much earlier and can appreciate contours and distance adequately. Such is not the case for those who become monocular during adult life. Skiing should also be proscribed to those who have undergone major eye surgery within three to six months.

Hockey

There are no prevailing standards for vision and visual fields for hockey. The National Hockey League, for the matter, has no policy related to visual standards. Most professional hockey teams check grossly the visual acuity and conduct a confrontation visual field. Players with a defect are sometimes referred to an ophthalmologist, but poor visual acuity or amblyopia is not a restriction for playing hockey. Some professional teams have higher visual standards than others and perform more refined testing. However, this would appear to be the exception. Of course, the puck is easy to identify, being dark on a bright white surface. Color vision is probably of greater importance since a player identifies teammates mainly by the color of their uniform. Playing hockey for pleasure call for no specific visual requirements; in fact, some very proficient professionals have had one amblyopic eye. Athletes who have strong ametropia should be encouraged to wear contact lenses which improve acuity and provide a better visual field. However, they should not induce a false sense of security, since they offer no protection.[4]

INJURIES

The prototypic victim of hockey-associated ocular injury in 1985 was an adult amateur, between 25 and 35 years of age, who played hockey once or twice a week, often to seek, rather than maintain physical fitness. Such an individual usually played hockey when tired, sometimes immediately after work, or late at night, when reflexes are impaired. Often, these adults return to hockey many years after having performed during their youth. In their childhood, they were not accustomed to wear a face protector nor a helmet; unfortunately, as adults, many fail to recognize the need for such protection. This type of player is, therefore, at risk. Should an eye injury occur, it will necessitate hospitalization in 30 percent of the cases, for one week or more. Late complications develop frequently and result in absence from work for weeks or even months with all the attending economic, familial, and social consequences.

The types of injuries most frequently encountered in skiing and hockey are peculiar to each discipline.

Hockey

The most frequent injury is induced by the hockey stick, mainly through high sticking, followed closely by the puck-related injuries.[4] The blade is seldom the case of an eye injury. Surveys done by the Canadian Ophthalmological Society, the Quebec Association of Ophthalmologists, and the Quebec Sports Safety Board (Régie de la sécurité dans les sports) have shown that hyphema is the most frequent eye injury (31.3%), followed by injuries to the lids and ocular adenexa.[5]

Hyphema

It is most important for the primary care physician to recognize hyphema or hemorrhage in the anterior chamber of the eye (Fig. 12-2). Immediate treatment should consist in restricting all physical activities and protecting the eye with a shield. The patient should then be referred to an ophthalmologist, since most of the time hospitalization will be required. Bleeding stems from rupture of an iris vessel of the major or minor arterial circle, and blood accumulates in the inferior portion of the anterior chamber. Vision is frequently reduced and the pupil is somewhat dilated. Treatment is still a matter of controversy among ophthalmologists, but what is unquestionable is that a recurrent hyphema is a most serious complication which might compromise the eye and, hence, calls for early detection. Generally, this secondary hemorrhage is rare and when it happens, it does so after three or four days. The hyphema can then be total (Fig. 12-3) and a sharp rise in the intraocular pressure is observed; this sometimes necessitates surgical treatment. This condition is known as the "Eight Ball Syndrome." One must bear in mind that even if the hyphema follows a favorable evolution, the traumatized eye is prone to late complication such as glaucoma or retinal detachment. For this reason, it is of utmost importance that the periphery of the fundus be checked after four weeks to detect a retinal dialysis or a peripheral retinal detachment that calls for urgent treatment. The player can resume activity in four weeks if the hyphema pursues an uneventful course.

Soft Tissue

Soft tissues injuries are often repaired in the emergency room, but close attention must be paid to those involving the margin of the lid and those located near the inner canthus. Such injuries, if not treated properly, can result in a lid notch causing chronic irritation or obstruction of the lacrimal drainage system. It is obviously very important to rule-out an injury to the eyeball itself. However, if there is a significant hematoma or edema of the lids, the examination should be performed with great care in the event that the lid's injury conceals a perforating injury of the eye.

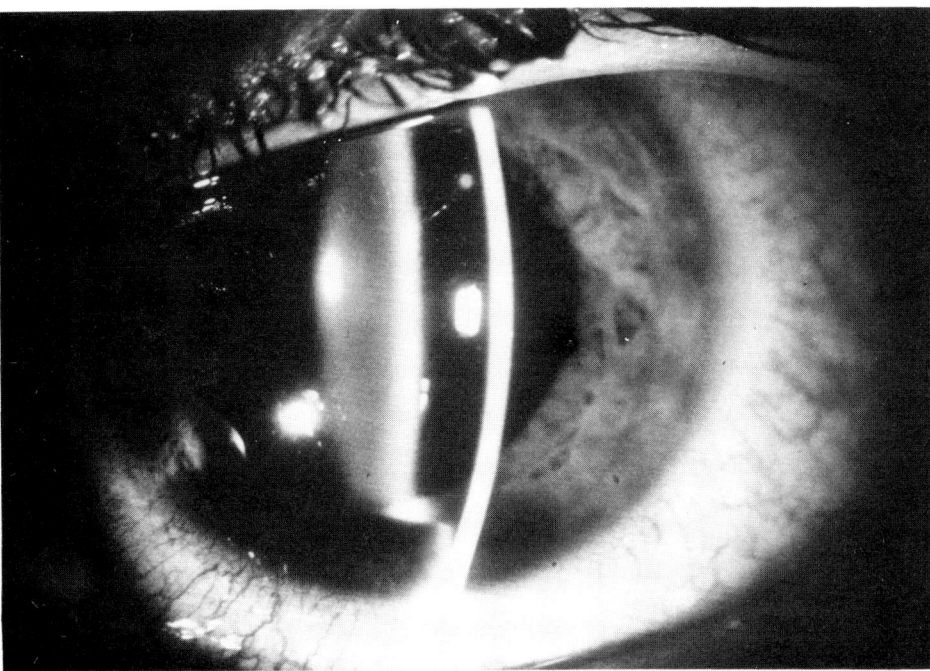

Figure 12-2. Hyphema or hemorrhage in the anterior chamber of the eye. The patient was a goaltender wearing molded face mask seen in figure 12-8.

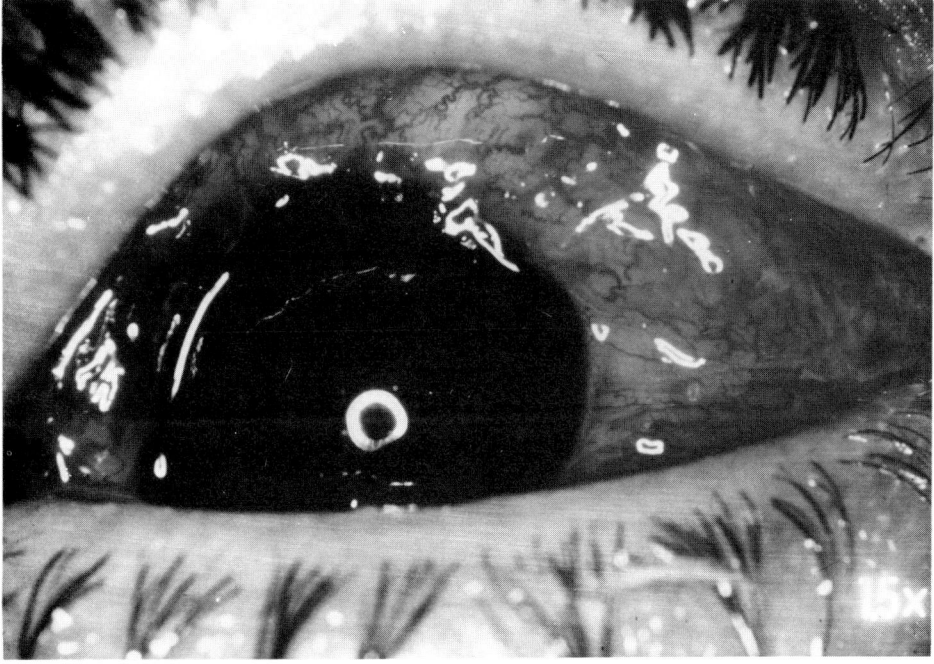

Figure 12-3. Total hyphema with secondary glaucoma, so-called "Eight Ball Syndrome."

Perforating Injuries

Sometimes ocular perforation is obvious (Fig. 12-4), but conjunctival hemorrhage or conjunctival edema can mask scleral rupture. In those cases, the examining physician can oftentimes, with aid of a flashlight, detect a shallowing of the anterior chamber or pupillary abnormalities such as anisocoria, pupillary irregularity, or pupillary retraction towards the wound. Emergency treatment is limited to a minimum of manipulation, topical antibiotics, and an eyeshield. Surgery is performed under general anesthesia with an operating microscope.

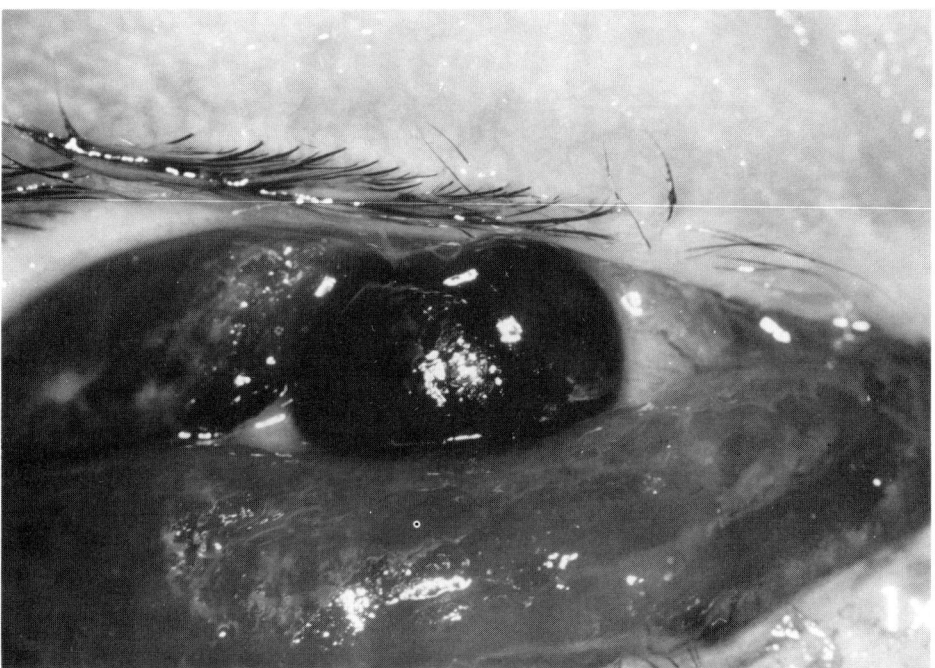

Figure 12-4. Perforating injury of the globe caused by a hockey stick; note the marked swelling of the conjunctival (chemosis) and hyphema.

Posterior Segment Injuries

Posterior segment injuries are many and can include vitreous hemorrhages, subretinal hemorrhages, choroidal rupture, retinal tear, and retinal detachment. It is important to remember that very often these potentially blinding injuries present without any obvious external sign of trauma. For this reason, it is important to perform a thorough funduscopic examination of an injured eye. Vitreous hemorrhages tend to reabsorb spontaneously. Vitrectomy is seldom necessary before six months. An echographic evaluation of the retina should be performed, and if a retinal detachment is suspected, earlier surgery should be contemplated.

Subretinal hemorrhages (Fig. 12-5) also reabsorb spontaneously and require no surgical intervention, although they may result in a damaging scar.

Choroidal rupture is often the result of a blunt trauma. Even though it may have a benign appearance (Fig. 12-6), such rupture may involve the macular area and reduce vision to 20/200 (6/60) or less. A subretinal neovascular membrane frequently develops, necessitating laser photocoagulation.

Retinal detachment is a serious consequence of posterior segment injuries and frequently requires major surgery. Because of damage to the vitreous body either directly or through hemorrhage, one is at risk for the development of proliferative vitreoretinopathy which may severely compromise the prognosis. Newer vitrectomy techniques have, however, improved the outlook. Even following a successful repair, the patient is usually not permitted to resume hockey playing.

Table 12-1

	NUMBER OF CASES	BLINDNESS	PERCENTAGE
All Sports	2 365	265	11,2%
Hockey	1 239	180	14,5%
Ski	10	6	60 %

Eye injuries secondary to sports (Canadian Ophthalmological Society—[1973 to July 1984]).

Late Complications

Trauma to the eye can give rise to late complications years later such as glaucoma, retinal detachment, or cataract. A study of 33 patients with retinal detachments secondary to hockey injuries treated over a period of 15 years at the Retina Clinic of Maisonneuve-Rosemont Hospital, has shown that the average interval between the accident and the preop examination had been three years, although the range extended from a few days to 29 years.[6]

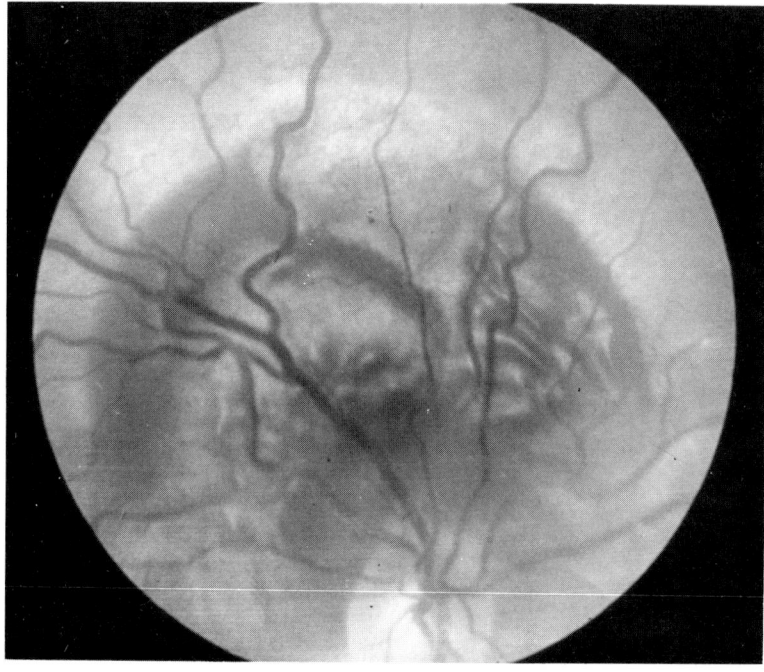

Figure 12-5. Subretinal hemorrhage around the optic disc caused by a puck.

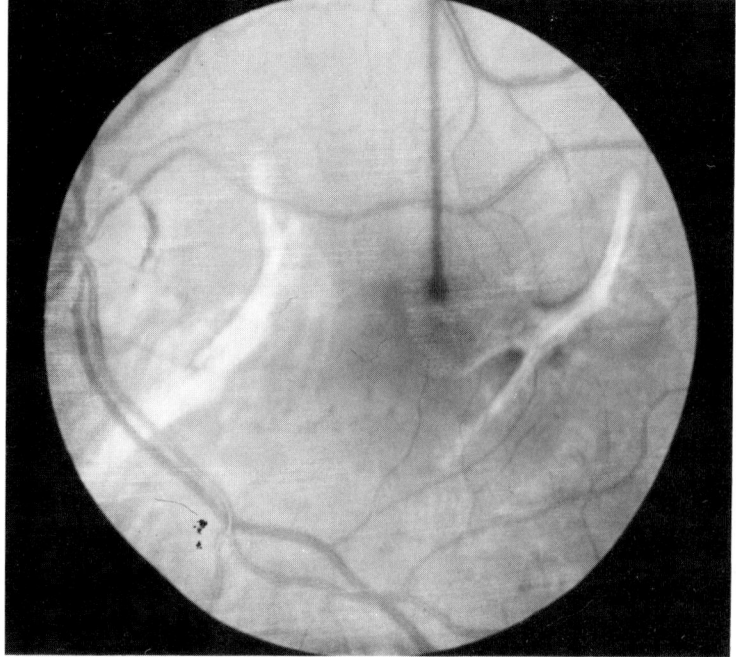

Figure 12-6. Cicatricial choroidal rupture reducing vision to 20/200 (6/60).

Skiing

Eye injuries to skiers, even though not as frequent, are of importance because of the high percentage of resulting severe handicap. (Table 12-1)

Snow Blindness

Ultraviolet keratitis, or snow blindness, was described in 1722 by St. Yves in individuals who had wandered in snow fields. Skiing at high altitude increases exposure to ultraviolet rays. Sunlight in the Alps contains between 5 and 6 percent of ultraviolet irradiation as compared to 1-2 percent in the tropics.[7] Thus, the quantity of ultraviolet irradiation reflected by the snow becomes important in instances of exposure for many hours. If a skier practices his sport on a nice sunny day, the cornea could receive a significant quantity of ultraviolet irradiation and keratitis could ensue. In such a case, the skier would experience at the end of the day or during the night, a burning sensation analogous to a multitude of small foreign bodies caused by epithelial cells injury and the exposure of nerve endings. Treatment consists of occlusion of the eye with an antibiotic ointment. Usually, the lesion subsides without sequelae within 24 hours.

Corneal Abrasion

The most frequent ocular injury in alpine skiing and cross-country skiing occurs when the eye strikes a tree branch. Most of the time, this trauma produces a superficial corneal erosion which heals with conventional treatment of occlusion. In some instances, such trauma can result, in the following months or even years, in a recurrent corneal erosion with its typical nocturnal or morning pain. Treatment of recurrent erosions may extend over many months and consists of an isotonic or hypertonic lubricating ointment (NaCl 5%).

Perforating Injuries

Following a fall while skiing, the eye may be hit by the ski edge or, more often, the ski pole. Avulsion of the optic nerve by the tip of a ski pole has been reported. We have also encountered conjunctival laceration, muscle transection, and/or corneoscleral perforation. Similar types of injuries can be produced by a T-bar.[8]

Posterior Segment Injuries

Serious posterior segment injuries include vitreous hemorrhage, retinal detachment, and choroidal rupture. The treatment, management, and prognosis are similar to corresponding injuries in hockey.

Broomball and Floor Hockey

The types of ocular injury which may be produced by accidents in broomball or floor hockey are similar to those incurred in ice hockey.

PREVENTION

Evolution of Eye Injuries Over the Past Decade

It was a shock to the ophthalmologists and the general community when we learned about ten years ago that during a single hockey season, approximately forty eyes had suffered blinding injuries and that the victims were mainly children in organized hockey. The Canadian Ophthalmological Society undertook, under the leadership of Dr. Thomas J. Pashby, during the 1974-75 season, a prospective study to quantitate hockey-associated ocular injuries. One-hundred-fourteen ophthalmologists reported 258 injuries (80% in organized hockey), which resulted in the functional loss of an eye in 42 instances. Victims were concentrated between the age of 11 and 15 years, and, in 63 percent of cases, the hockey stick was the direct cause of injury.[9]

It then became obvious that something had to be done to reduce this carnage. Rule changes were introduced to eliminate high sticking and, above all, the face protector was designed, the use of which has become more widespread. Two Canadian cities, Brampton, Ontario, and Outremont, Quebec, rapidly indicated the path to follow by making it mandatory that all young hockey players wear a face protector. The following year this preventive measure was imposed upon all players of minor hockey in Canada (1976-77). Since then, we have seen an almost total disappearance of ocular injuries in young players.

In the United States, during the seventies, Dr. Paul F. Vinger, impressed by the number of ocular injuries resulting from hockey, formed a committee to study the proble of ocular injuries resulting from sports.[10] In 1974, the committee report suggested that facial protection be mandatory and, in a preliminary study, defined the criteria for effective facial protection. A USA-Canada collaboration then followed in order to attain the goal of eliminating eye injuries for all hockey players, whether in Canada or in the United States. In amateur hockey leagues, the requirement for a face mask was made mandatory during the 1976-77 season for the 400,000 hockey players of the Amateur Hockey Association of the United States. In 1980, the report from the American Medical Association urged that "all amateur, high school, and college hockey programs throughout the nation require the use of hockey face masks."[10]

Nevertheless, despite those measures and irrefutable efficacy of the face protector (which continues to reflect design improvements), recent statistics show that hockey remains an important cause of ocular injuries in sports; in Canada, hockey tops the list. The cumulative data of the Canadian Ophthalmological Society show that of 2,365 injuries reported to the Society as of July 1st 1984, 1,239 were hockey-related, of which 14.5 percent led to blindness (Table 12-1). This table further indicates that ski injuries are much less frequently reported, but should be considered as an important problem since 60 percent of the reported injuries were blinding. A survey in Quebec between May, 1982 and June, 1984[6] showed that of 460 sport-associated eye injuries, 124 or 27.4 percent were secondary to hockey. This figure was comparable to a previous study.[11]

How is it possible that since we have almost completely eliminated eye injuries in youngsters, hockey continues to account for about 30 percent of sport-associated eye injuries in Canada? There are several plausible reasons. First, the early statistics obtained on hockey injuries were probably incomplete and underestimated the magnitude of the problem. Second, the popularity of hockey has been increasing among amateur adults in the northern United States and Canada. Since these amateurs are not required to wear a face protector, many neglect to do so.

In 1980, Dr. Vinger[12] estimated that a certified face protector could reduce by over 90 percent the number of face injuries, thus preventing approximately 70,000 injuries to Americans, representing an approximate economy of $10,000,000.00 to society. It is regrettable that this security measure has not been made obligatory, at least in amateur sports. For this reason, our recent publicity has been directed to this type of hockey player (Fig. 12-7).

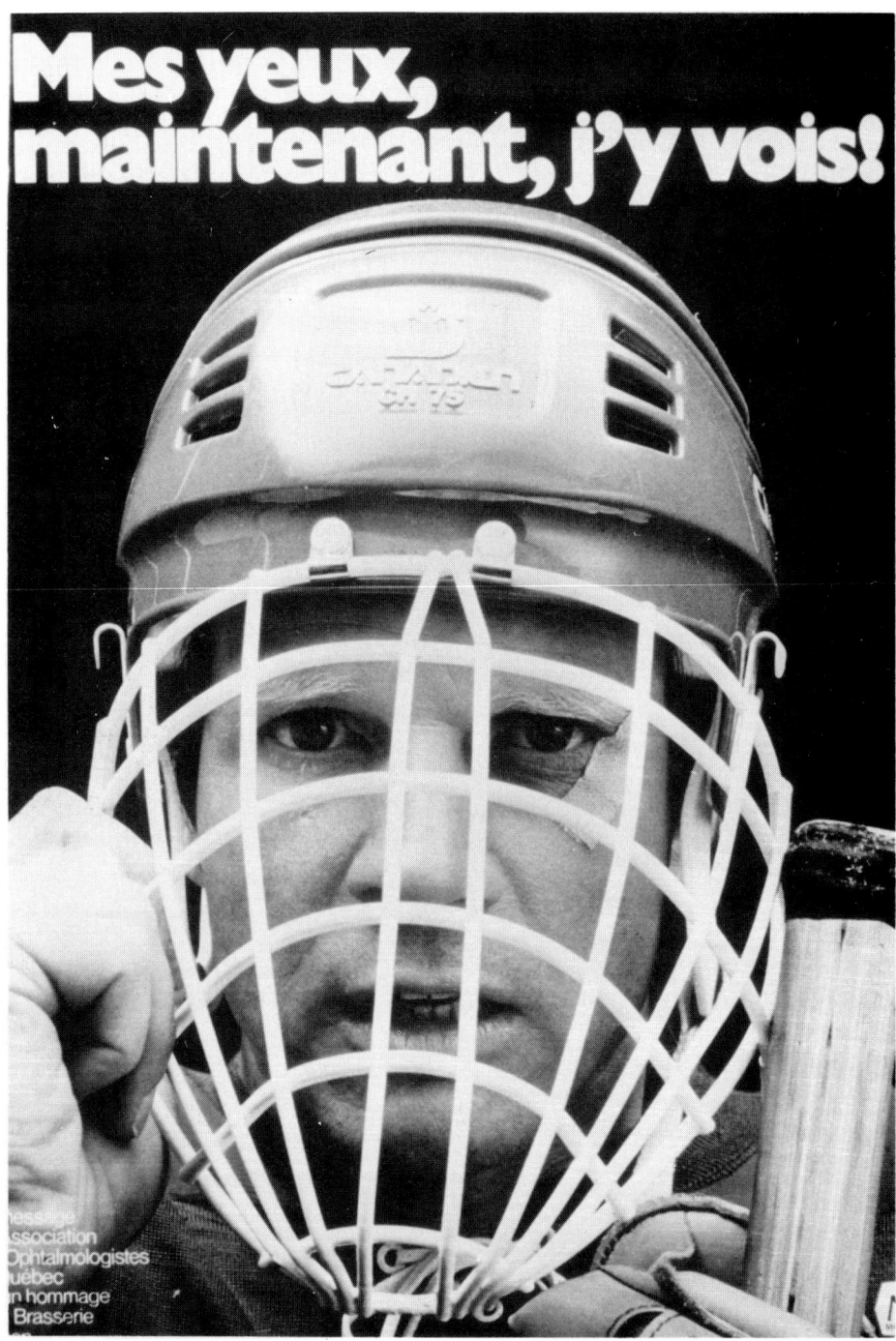

Figure 12-7. Poster distributed by the "Association des Ophtalmologistes du Quebec" promoting eye safety in hockey.

Goalers

Jacques Plante, formerly of the Montreal Canadians, was a pioneer in the early sixties when he popularized the use of a molded face mask for goalers. Nevertheless, even though the idea was excellent, it was realized later that his type of protector for goalers was inadequate. Indeed, the Canadian Ophthalmological Society has, in its records, approximately a dozen eye injuries sustained by goalers wearing this type of molded face mask, a fact which can be easily understood by referral to Figure 12-8. Most goalers today wear a wire mesh face protector instead of molded mask, thus preventing any possibility for the introduction of the puck or end of a hockey stick.

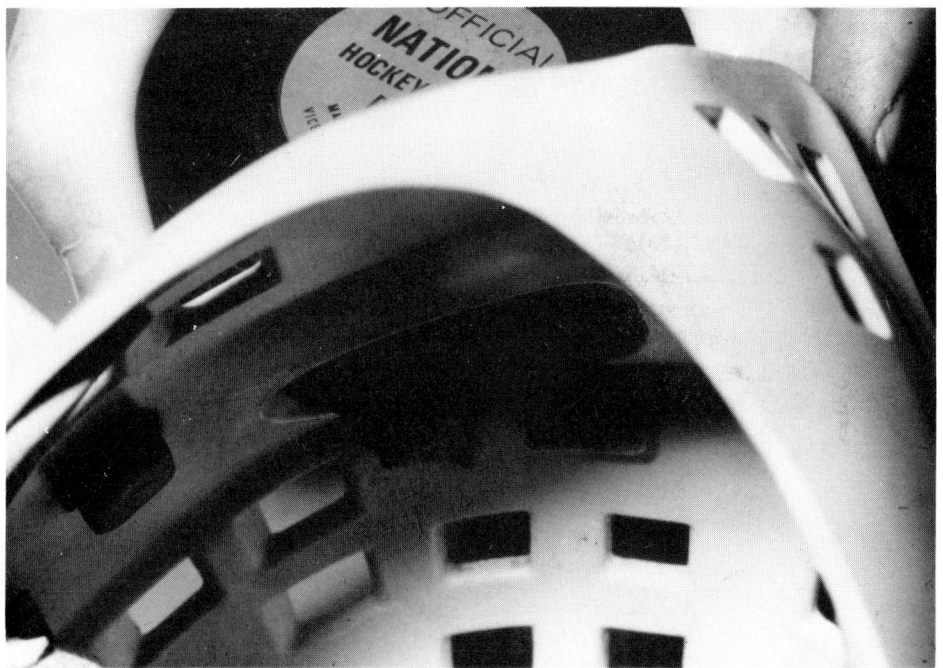

Figure 12-8. Molded face mask for goaltenders. An ocular injury can occur when the puck passes through an opening at the eye level.

Referees

We are aware of at least two injuries suffered by hockey referees, one of which was very serious. It has been suggested that hockey referees be required to wear a face protector covering at least the superior part of the face (Fig. 12-9). This protector would prevent most eye injuries without impediment to the use of the whistle.

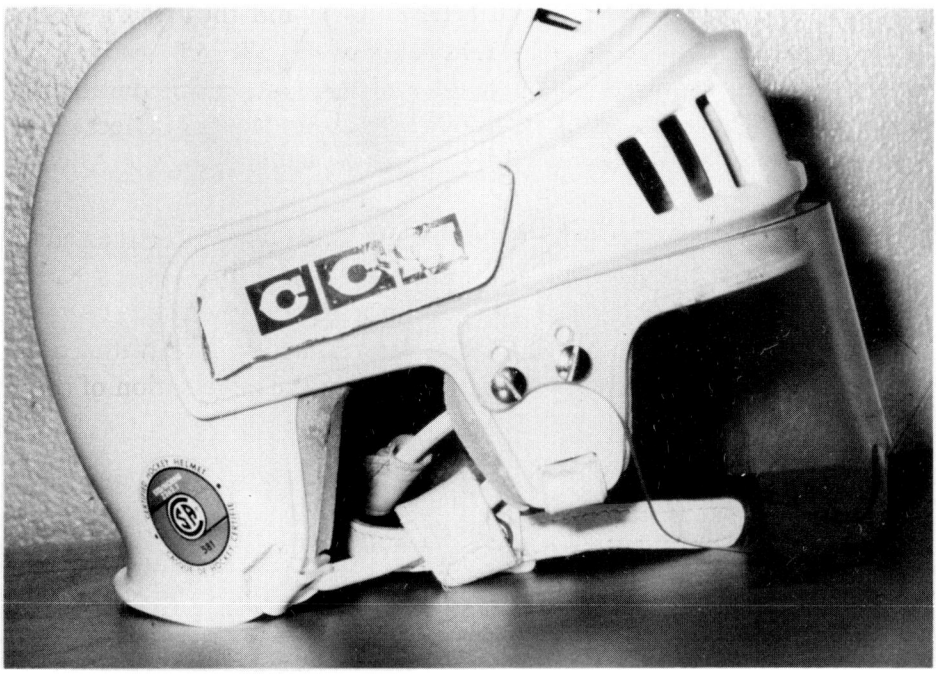

Figure 12-9. Polycarbonate visor covering the superior part of the face, recommended for referees, but not players.

Spectators

Injuries suffered by spectators at a hockey game are rarely reported, but nevertheless, those who have attended such game know that a spectator sometimes leaves his seat suffering from a face injury. It is, thus, important that standards for glass protectors around the rink be established and respected.

Hockey Face Protector

The hockey face protector is designed to avoid injury to the eye, orbital area, and face by the hockey stick, puck, or any other possible mechanism. It is relatively easy to adapt a face protector to most hockey helmets. Ideally, the protector should not interfere with vision, provide a maximum of protection, and resist major impacts, such as a puck travelling at more than a 100 miles/hour.[13] Presently, two models are available: the wire-mesh type and the polycarbonate type. Both are approved by the Canadian Standard Association (C.S.A.), the Hockey

Equipment Certification Council (H.E.C.C.), and the American Society for Testing Materials (A.S.T.M.). As of the 1985-86 season, face protectors were required for all players of the National Federation of States High School Association. Similar requirements take effect in the season 1986-87 for players in the National Collegiate Athletic Association.[14]

The wire mesh protector is very effective in protecting against sticks or pucks, yet some players feel some kind of a visual impediment by the wire. The more closely apposed the wire, the greater the protection and sense of visual impairment. It has been determined that the distance between wires should be small enough to prevent the penetration of tip of the stick (Fig. 12-10).

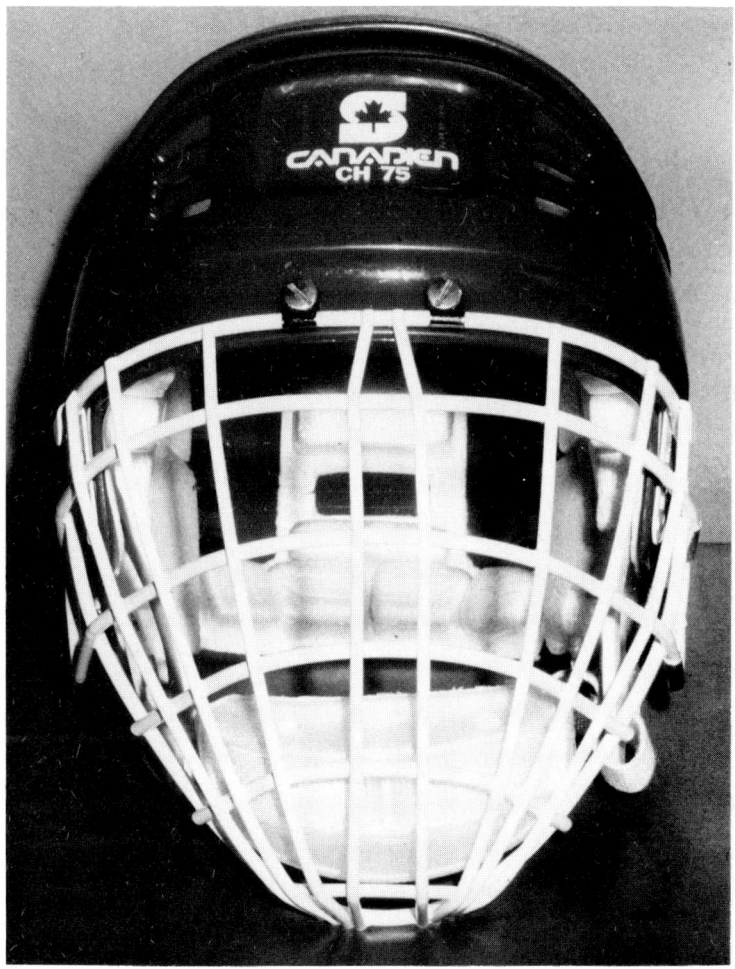

Figure 12-10. Wire mesh face protector.

The plastic guard is made from polycarbonate and should cover the whole face. This specially treated polycarbonate, is resistant to scratches and has an interior coating against fogging (Fig. 12-11). This treated polycarbonate is 9 times more resistant to impact than before treatment and is 30 times more resistant than hardened glass. While the face mask wire mesh might give the player a sense of impaired vision, visual field testing by the authors has not shown any limitation of the peripheral field at the Goldman perimeter. There is no difference in the field of vision between the wire mesh, the plastic visor or without any face protector. With the aid of the computerized visual field testing (Octopus 500), programs 24, 36, and 38 have not shown any significant impediments except for a very small relative inferior scotoma with the wire mesh guard (Fig. 12-12 and 12-13).

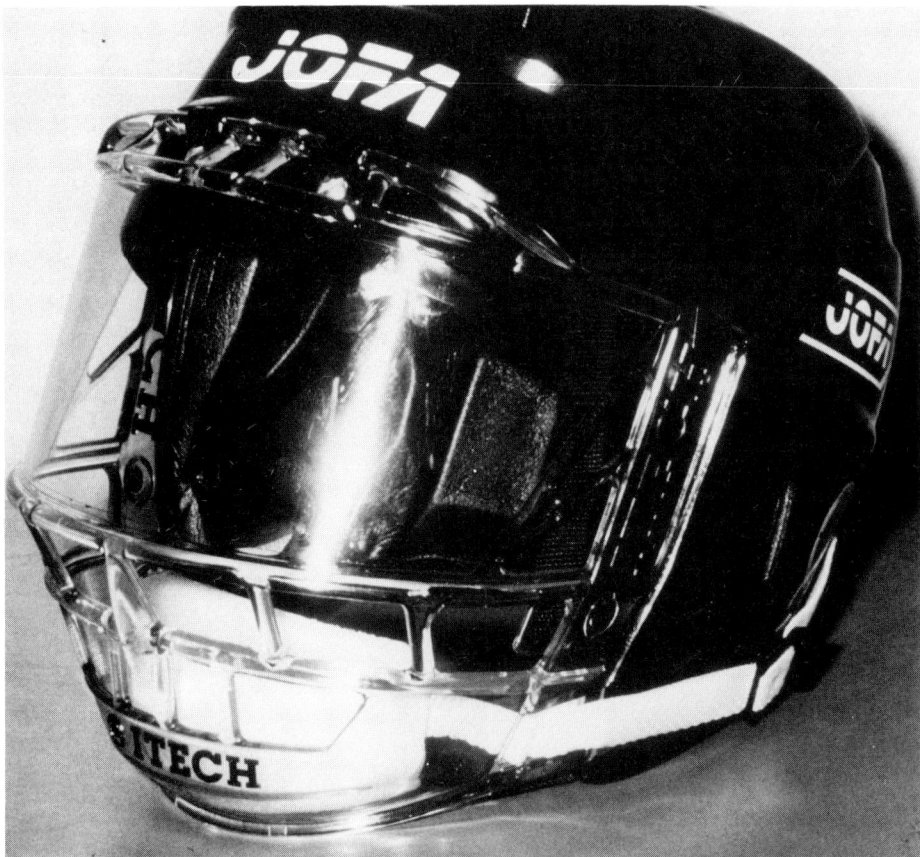

Figure 12-11. Polycarbonate face protector.

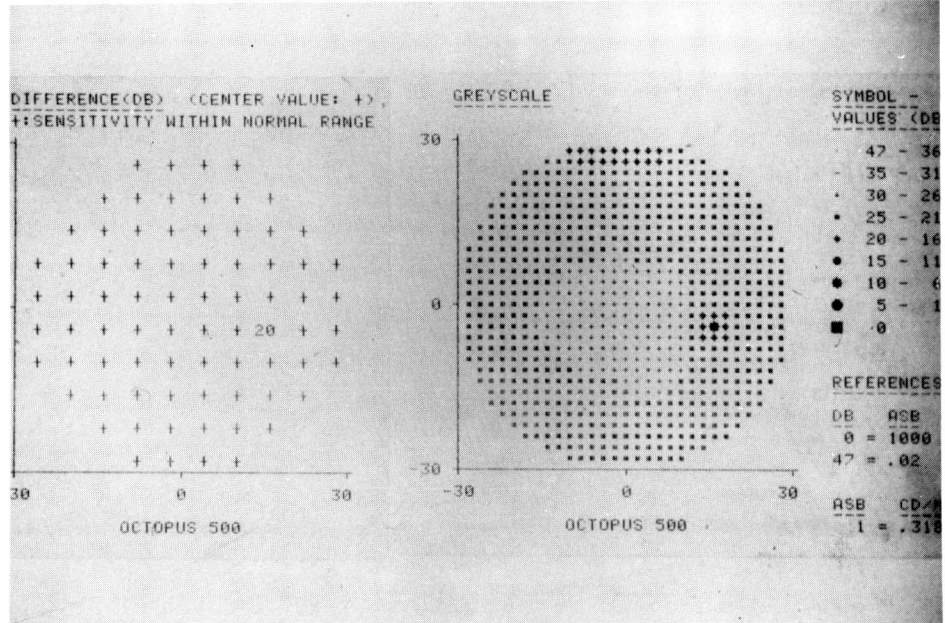

Figure 12-12. Computerized visual field (program 36, Octopus 500) performed in an individual wearing a full-face polycarbonate protector shows no scotoma.

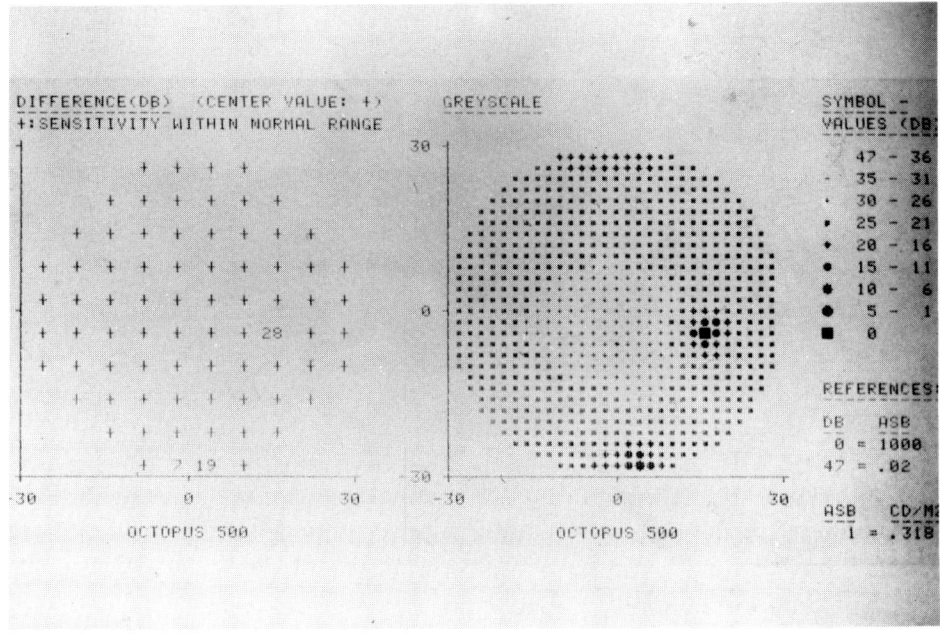

Figure 12-13. Computerized visual field (program 36, Ocotpus 500) performed in an individual wearing a wire mesh mask; note the small relative inferior scotoma.

Ski Goggles

A good ski goggle should offer some protection against mechanical and optical interferences. Many models currently available (Fig. 12-14) are strong enough to deviate the tip of a ski pole, the tip of the ski or the branch of a tree in order to prevent ocular injuries.

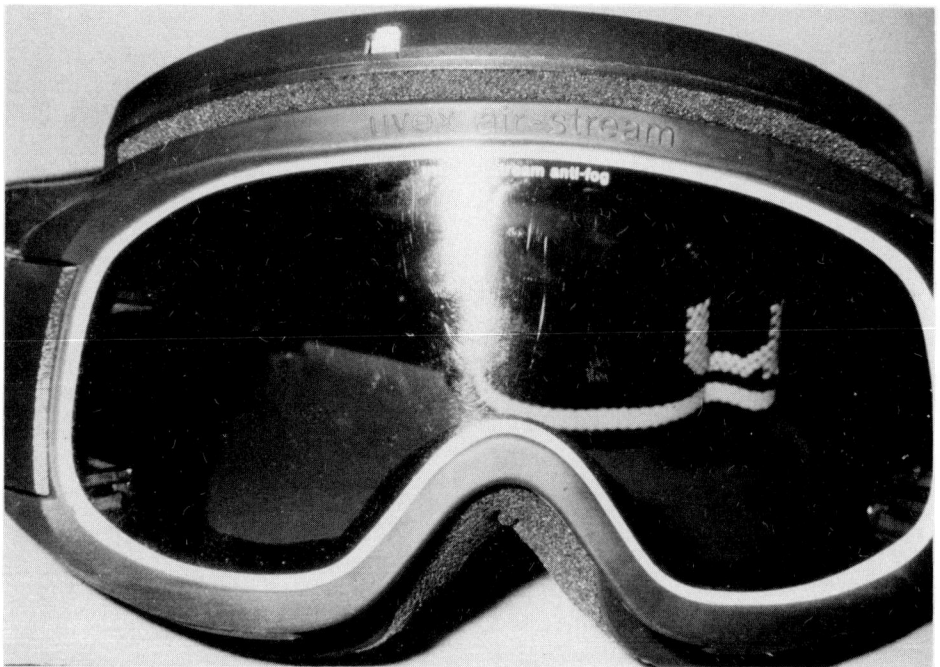

Figure 12-14. Ski goggles.

Snow blindness is preventable by wearing an antiultraviolet lens capable of elimination rays from 300 to 470 nanometers in length. Some models can accept optical prescription up to 8 diopters for the sphere and 5 diopters in cylinder. Many skiers operated for cataract should wear special lens against ultraviolet rays because it is well-established that such patients can incur retinal problems if exposed to ultraviolet rays which, in the past, were filtered by their own lens.

In downhill skiing, the wind and cold might increase the quantity of tears, making vision somewhat blurred and decreasing the perception of moguls. Many ski goggles are wide enough to offer full field of vision without interference and many have a double lens antifog property. Some models are wider and can be worn over a pair of eyeglasses (Fig. 12-15).

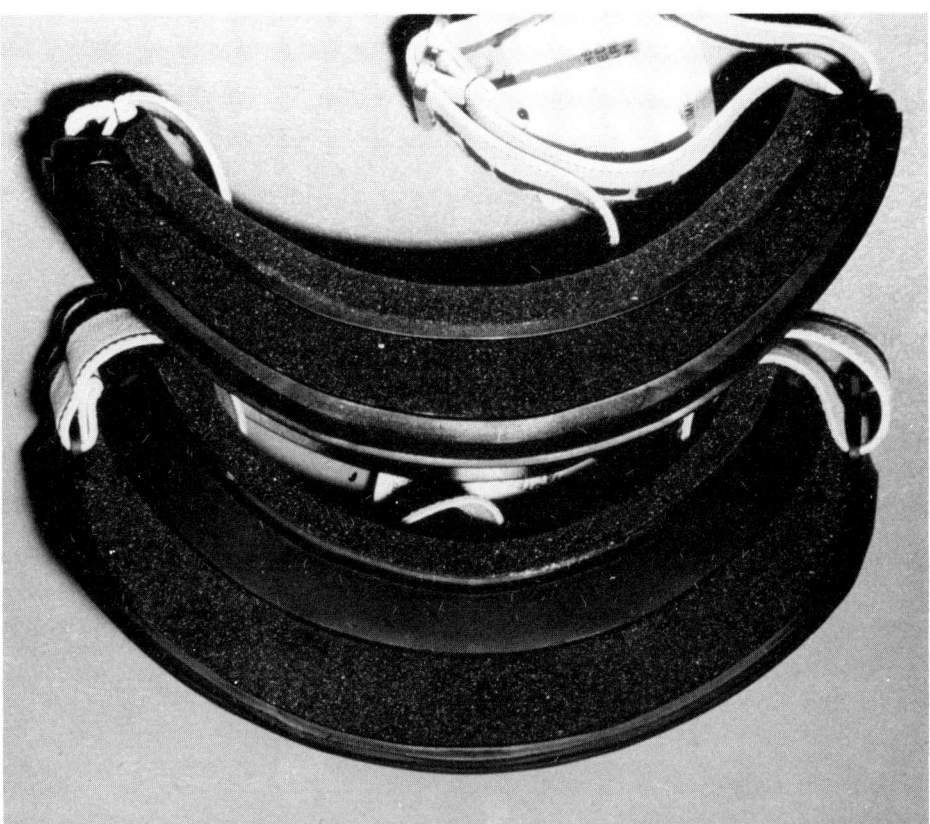

Figure 12-15. Some models of ski goggles can be worn over a pair of eyeglasses.

The contact lens by itself does not offer any protection, but can improve vision by increasing the visal field and visual acuity and by decreasing or eliminating some aberrations in patients with strong ametropia.

CONCLUSION

"Prevention is better than the best treatment." This should be and is applicable to the skier and hockey player. During the last ten years, substantial progress toward the prevention of ocular injuries has been made in sports, particularly hockey. Twenty-five years ago, even the goalers wore no protective device over the face and head. Effective hockey face protectors and ski goggles now exist. Physicians and ophthalmologists should be aware that protection is available for players. They have a responsibility to educate the public regarding prevention of ocular or face trauma. As more youngsters come to accept as normal facial protectors, one may anticipate the day wherein participants at all levels of hockey will feel comfortable and secure with such protection.

REFERENCES

1. Chevaleraud, J.P.: Oeil et Sports, Masson, Paris, 1983.
2. Perchél G. et Chevaleraud J.P.: Aspects ophtalmologiques du ski de compétition, *Bull. Med. Ski, Mai,* 1969.
3. Wiedman, M.: Nouvelle recherche oculaire au Mont Everst, *Bull. Med. Soc. Fr. Opht.,* 86, pp. 201-207, 1973.
4. Little, J.M.: Blessures oculaires au hockey, principales causes et prévention, *L'Actualité médicale,* pp. 46-48, Octobre 8, 1984.
5. Les blessures oculaires dans le sport au Québec—Étude de la Régie de la Sécurité dans les sports et de l'Association des Ophtalmologistes du Québec, Publication du Gouvernement du Québec, Février, 1985.
6. Antaki, S., Labelle, P., Dumas, J.: "Retinal Detachment following Hockey Injury, *Canadian Medical Association, J. 117:* 245, 1977.
7. Duke-Elder: "System of Ophthalmology, vol. XIV, Injuries, part II, Henry Kimpton, 1972.
8. Amyot, M.: L'oeil et le ski, condition de'exposition et protection, *L'Actualité médicale,* vol. 5, no. 20, pp. 37-39, Octobre 8, 1984.
9. Pashby, T.J., Pashby, R.C., Chisholm, L.D.J., Crawford, J.S.: "Eye Injuries in Canadian Hockey," *Canadian Medical Association. J 113:* 663, 1975.
10. Vinger, P.F.: Appendix, "Eye and Face Protection for United States Hockey Players," *A. Chronology Intern. Ophthalm. Clinics,* Little, Brown, vol. 21, no. 4, pp. 83-86, 1981.
11. Rousseau, A.P.: *Ocular Trauma in Sports—Ocular Trauma,* H.M. Freeman Ed., section IX, ch. 36, pp. 353-361, Appleton Century Crofts, 1979.
12. Vinger, P.F.: "Sports Eye Injuries, A Preventable Disease," *Ophthalmol.,* 88, no. 2, pp. 108-133, 1981.
13. Vinger, P.F., "Principles of Protection," *Intern. Ophthalm. Clinics,* Little, Brown, vol. 21, no. 4, pp. 149-161, 1981.
14. The Physician and Sports Medicine, "Hockey Face Guards Required for 1985-86," vol. 13, no. 1, p. 29, Jan. 1985.

CHAPTER 13

SPORTS EYE INJURIES: FIRST AID AND PREVENTION

GEORGE S. ELLIS, Jr.

APPROXIMATELY two million eye injuries occur in the United States annually, 90 percent of which could be prevented.[1] Eye injuries are the fourth most common cause of visual loss in persons under the age of 45.

In our health conscious society, more and more people are taking an active part in sports. While the overall general health of our population is improving, the incidence of sports-related injuries continues to be high. According to the National Society to Prevent Blindness, approximately 40,000 sports-related eye injuries are treated each year in hospital emergency rooms. This number represents only a portion of the estimated 100,000 sports eye injuries that occur annually. Unfortunately, approximately 25,000 of these progress to serious and potentially sight-damaging complications.

In the United States, racquet sports cause almost one-third of all sports-related eye injuries to athletes between the ages of 25 and 65, while baseball is the most common cause of eye injury in children ages 5 to 15. In Canada, hockey accounts for about 50 percent of sports-related eye injuries.

Sports-related eye injuries may be ameliorated by first aid and subsequent definitive treatment, but prevention is unquestionably more effective in reducing serious visual consequences. The generic item of protective gear is the face guard, which has been adapted to the individual requirements of various sports. As described in Dr. Rousseau's chapter on winter sports, the Canadian Ophthalmological Society reported-the virtual elimination of ocular injuries in young hockey players ages 11 to 15 years in the year after the wearing of effective face protectors became mandatory. Before this, the functional loss of an eye had been associated with approximately 42 injuries in children in this group.

Whether or not to participate at all is of less impact statistically, but of enormous individual significance. Preparticipation eye screening and referral should help to identify those people at high risk because of preexisting ocular conditions. A physician who is knowledgeable about the risks of a given sport and conversant with the history and clinical status of the prospective athlete can help to decide if participation is worth the risk.

When a sports-related ocular injury occurs, someone on the scene must immediately evaluate the severity of the problem, and triage the patient to the appropriate level of care. First aid personnel can provide definitive treatment for some minor injuries; the depth and breadth of the first aid administered depends on their experience and training. Serious injuries should be referred to a medical eye physician (ophthalmologist). It is always best to err on the side of caution; for the sake of the athlete's vision, it is always safer to overdiagnose and over-refer. This chapter emphasizes the prevention and first aid of sports-related ocular injuries, as well as the signs and symptoms of more serious problems for which ophthalmological assistance should be sought.

PREVENTION

Previous Ocular Injury or Surgery

Anyone who has had previous eye surgery or injury should consult an ophthalmologist prior to engaging in any new sport. This recommendation is particularly true for a person who has had a retinal detachment or has undergone radial keratotomy (RK) for nearsightedness (myopia). Patients who have large degrees of nearsightedness (high myopia) have an increased risk of retinal detachment whether or not RK has been performed. Even noncontact sports, such as jogging, may cause retinal detachments in such people.

A special situation exists with prospective athletes who have only one functional eye, i.e., the vision in the worse eye is 20/200 or less, while the better eye sees normally. This poor vision (20/200) is the upper limit of legal blindness. Some persons have decreased function if their only eye sees less than 20/40 (the usual limit for a driver's license). Such individuals are at risk of losing their only eye to injury during sports activities. They must be made aware not only of the risks of injury, but also of the protective devices available. At a minimum, the one-eyed athlete should use an eye protector for all and any sports.

Protective Gear

Protective eye wear has been shown to be extraordinarily effective in preventing sport injuries.[2] The vast majority of ocular injuries occurring during sport activities could probably be prevented if proper protective eye wear were used. Important considerations include the lens material, the nose pads, which should be an integral part of the frame, and the bridge of the frame across the nose, which should be quite strong. A lengthy description of various protective equipment is found in Chapter 2.

Many different eye protectors and helmets have been designed, and standards for specific sports may be available from any of several organizations. The American National Standards Institute, the American Society for Testing in Materials, and the Canadian Standards Association are organizations that may be able to provide current standards for each sport. Table 13-1 summarizes protective equipment available for various sports.

Table 13-1
RISK FACTORS AND PROTECTIVE GEAR FOR VARIOUS SPORTS

Sport	Recommended Protector	Relative Risk Factor 1 (Low); 10 (High)
Auto Racing	Helmet with separate eye protector	10
Baseball (Catcher, Umpire)	Full-face protector	7
Baseball (fielders)	Sport eye protector	7
Basketball	Sport eye protector	7
Boxing	Helmet only	10
Cross-Country Skiing	Sport eye protector	3
Cycling	Helmet with separate eye protector	3
Fencing	Full-face protector	1
Fishing	Eye Glasses	3
Football	Total head protector	5
Golf	Sport eye protector	3

(continued)

Sport	Recommended Protector	Relative Risk Factor 1 (Low); 10 (High)
Hockey	Total head protector	10
Horseback Riding/Polo	Helmet with separate eye protector	5
Jogging/Running	Sport eye protector	1
Lacrosse	Total head protector	10
Racquetball/Squash	Sport eye protector, Class II or III	9
Ski Racing	Helmet with separate eye protector	3
Snow Mobiling	Helmet with separate eye protector	3
Soccer	Sport eye protector	5
Softball	Sport eye protector	7
Swimming	Sport eye protector	1
Tennis	Sport eye protector	7

PREPARTICIPATION SCREENING

An eye examination should be performed before the prospective athlete undertakes a new sport activity. The preparticipation examination may help to uncover any existing ocular conditions that require a full medical evaluation and also provide a baseline with which postinjury screening can be compared. The preparticipation examination should include a medical history focused on previous eye diseases, injuries or surgery, as well as the testing of visual acuity (central vision), visual field (peripheral vision), the pupils and eye movement.

History

The prospective athlete should be asked the following questions specifically: whether he or she wears glasses (especially thick ones) or contact lenses; whether he or she has had surgery for cataract, retinal detachment, or nearsightedness (radial keratotomy), or a corneal transplant; and whether he or she has ever had a cut, bruise, or bleeding of the eye.

The Eye Examination

In the absence of a previous history of eye injury or surgery the preparticipation screening examination can be performed by trained first aid or paramedical personnel. The components of the eye examination are described below.

Visual Acuity

To test visual acuity, you will need an eye chart. A distance eye chart is usually placed 20 feet from the subject, while a near vision chart is held 14 inches from the eyes. If the prospective athlete cannot read the 20/40 line with each eye tested individually, then he or she should see an ophthalmologist for a detailed examination. For baseline information, it is desirable to test vision at both distance and near.

Visual Fields

Confrontation visual fields test peripheral or side vision. In essence, the examiner is comparing his/her own field of side vision to that of the athlete. Again, each eye is tested independently. The examiner compares the athlete's right eye with the examiner's left eye, and vice versa. To perform the test, the examiner sits facing the athlete, about 3-4 feet apart. The examiner places his/her hand half-way between the two of them. The hand is then moved to the side (or up or down), outside the examiner's field of vision, while the examiner's open eye continues to look at the eye being tested. The athlete should stare at the examiner's open eye. As the examiner slowly brings his hand back toward his field of view, the athlete indicates when he can first see the examiner's fingers. This test should be repeated in all four quadrants of the visual field for each eye.

Pupils

The pupils should also be tested with a flashlight or penlight. While the athlete is looking at a distance, the examiner shines the light into one eye. The reaction of the pupil is observed. Ideally, the screener should note the size and shape of the pupil before and after illumination and the briskness of the constrictions. The light can be moved away and then back to the eye several times as necessary. Subsequently, the other eye should be evaluated.

After the shape, size, and reactivity of each pupil are noted, a comparison between pupils is helpful. Swing the flashlight from eye to eye and note if the pupils constrict or dilate as the eye is illuminated. A pupil that dilates when illuminated with the swinging flashlight test may indicate severe abnormality and require expert evaluation.

Other findings requiring ophthalmological evaluation include a difference in size or reactivity of the pupils. Also, any irregularity in shape (normal pupils are round) should be cause for referral.

Eye Movements

Ocular motility is grossly tested by asking the athlete to look right and left and up and down. The eyes should move in all directions together. In the extremes of horizontal gaze, no white should be seen between the corner of the eyelid and the iris. The penlight may be used to create a light reflex on each cornea. The athlete should look directly at the penlight, which is held directly in front of the examiner. The corneal light reflexes should be symmetrical with respect to the pupils. This means that the reflex of the light should appear in the same location in each eye—both may be central or both slightly nasal, etc.

POSTINJURY SCREENING

The postinjury history is focused on incidents immediately surrounding the accident. The circumstances of the injury should be fully documented if possible. Did something fly into the eye? Was the athlete poked? An eye examination should be performed as described above.

Often at the time of injury, only near vision can be evaluated. The near vision card in the first-aid kit is valuable in this regard. Remember to test each eye separately, while being sure that the untested eye is completely occluded. An injured athlete unable to clear his or her blurred vision with blinking should be treated as a medical emergency and should be examined immediately in a hospital emergency room or by an ophthalmologist.

In the visual fields test, if the examiner notices his own fingers within his field of view significantly before the athlete reports seeing the fingers, it should be considered a medical emergency and the athlete should be examined by an ophthalmologist. Remember to repeat the test in all four quadrants of the visual field for each eye.

When the pupils are tested with a flashlight or penlight, any irregularity or abnormality of one or both pupils is cause for alarm. Pupil abnormalities (see section on pupils) are also a medical emergency.

Both eyes should move the same amount in all directions. When looking to the far left or right, the corner (angle) of the eyelids should meet the corneal-scleral junction. Each eye should move the same amount up or down. The light reflex created by the penlight can help in judging the position of the eyes.

If one eye does not move as far as the other in any direction, an expert evaluation should be obtained.

THE EMERGENCY EYE KIT

Table 13-2
EMERGENCY EYE CARE KIT

Type	Components
Basic	1) Emergency phone numbers (emergency rooms, ophthalmologists) 2) Near vision card, distance vision card 3) Small mirror, to look for lost contact lens 4) Suction cup to remove dislodged hard contact lens 5) Squeeze bottle for fluid to irrigate conjunctival foreign body 6) Sterile cotton swabs 7) Sterile strips to close the skin 8) Penlight 9) Oval eye pads (sterile) 10) Tape 11) Hard shields 12) Empty contact lens case
Advanced (To be used by physician only)	1) Anesthetic eye drops (Proparacaine) 2) Antibiotic eye drop (Neosporin) 3) Antibiotic eye ointment (10% Sodium Sulamyd) 4) Fluorescein strip

Contents

The contents of the typical emergency eye kit are listed in Table 13-2. Most of the items can be used by first aid personnel, but some are reserved for use by a physician. The utility of the various components is as follows:

The *vision cards* and *penlight* are used in the ocular examination described in detail above.

The *phone numbers* are often quite useful when, in the excitement of the emergency, it becomes necessary to contact the person or agency to whom the injured athlete is being referred.

A *small mirror* is useful when a contact lens is dislodged. Often the athlete can quickly locate the contact lens if such a mirror is available. By applying gentle pressure to the contact lens through the eyelid, it is often possible to correctly position a dislodged hard contact lens. If repositioning is unsuccessful, then the *small suction cup* (available from contact lens dispensers) is very helpful in removing the contact. Soft contact lenses are more easily wiped out with a *cotton swab*.

The *squeeze bottle* may be used with fluid (water, saline, etc.) to create a stream directed toward a foreign body located over the white of the eye. Nothing should be instilled in an eye in which you suspect that the eyeball is not intact.

If you suspect that the globe has been cut open, either on the sclera or cornea, then the eye should be protected with an *eye shield* taped from the forehead toward the ear. Do not apply a pad or medicine.

Anesthetic drops should not be used by other than a physician. Such drops should never be used to allow an injured athlete to resume participation in the sport.

Useful Techniques

Taping an *eye pad* or *eye shield* is an important skill. With a pad, the eye should be closed by the athlete before application as the surface of the pad will scratch the cornea if the lids are open. With a shield, the eye may be open or closed. The tape should be applied from the center of the forehead (glabella) toward the lower lobe of the ear (tragus of the mandible). Taping in this orientation will allow opening and closing of the mouth without dislodging the pad or shield. A paper drinking cup (or bottom half) may be substituted if a shield is unavailable.

Everting the upper eyelid is a technique worth knowing.[3] The basic concept is to fold the upper eyelid backwards on itself, such that the lashes are closer to the eyebrow. To perform this maneuver, one needs an instrument, such as a sterile cotton swab, and one's index finger and thumb. The examiner asks the patient to look down and then grasps the lashes of the upper lid, pulling them further down and out, away from the eye. The cotton swab is placed on the outside of the lid, at the level of the lid crease. The eyelashes are folded upwards, over the cotton swab, such that the pink conjunctiva lining the inside of the eyelid (tarsus) becomes visible. At this point, usually a conjunctival foreign body or dislodged contact lens can be located. The eyelid is returned to its normal position by asking the patient to look up and blink.

DISPOSITION OF OCULAR INJURIES

When an ocular injury has taken place, a decision must be made as to the nature and seriousness of the injury. Minor injuries can be treated by the person administering the first aid. More serious injuries should be referred to the care of the nearest ophthalmologist or emergency room. The most serious type of injury, a chemical burn, requires immediate and specific emergency therapy at the scene, followed by transfer to an emergency room. Some of the types of problems are described below, with suggestions for appropriate first aid approaches and recommendations for referral as needed.

Injuries Treatable by First Aid Personnel

Lost or Dislodged Contact Lens

Soft contact lenses are rarely dislodged, but when they are, vision is suddenly decreased. Inspection beneath the upper and lower eyelids will usually disclose the location of the contact lens. Experienced physicians may try a drop of Proparacaine, a topical anesthetic, followed by a gentle wipe with a sterile cotton tip applicator beneath both the upper and lower lids, in the attempt to locate the lens. Placing fluorescein inside the lid will permanently discolor the contact lens.

If a hard contact lens is dislodged, and the athlete cannot locate it using the small mirror included in the emergency eye kit, the first-aid giver may have to evert the upper lid. To move the lens back onto the cornea, gentle pressure may be applied through the closed eyelid. Sometimes a strong squeeze of fluid from the plastic squeeze bottle may help to dislodge a contact lens that is stuck to the conjunctiva. If the contact lens persistently adheres to the conjunctiva, then the small suction cup may be applied to the hard contact lens in order to lift it from the eye.

Conjunctival Foreign Body

A foreign body located on the conjunctiva is one of the more common problems that a first-aid person can immediately treat, allowing the athlete to return to the action. Usually the athlete complains that something has flown into his/her eye, and there is pain and tearing. Often there is continued blinking and a feeling of scratchiness. With continued scratching and blinking, a corneal abrasion may occur, leading to a more severe problem.

The first step is to locate the foreign body. This can be done by inspecting the white portion of the athlete's eye using the penlight. Have the athlete look in all directions, and if the foreign body is located on the white of the eye, it often can be irrigated off with a gentle burst of fluid from the squeeze bottle. Occasionally, a sterile cotton swab may be used to wipe away the foreign body. A foreign body located under the upper eyelid may be removed by using the lower eyelashes to brush the inside of the upper eyelid. The examiner should pull the upper eyelashes, such that the upper lid covers the skin of the lower eyelid. When the eye is opened, the lower eyelid lashes will attempt to clean the upper eyelid conjunctiva. If this is unsuccessful, then the upper eyelid may be everted as described above. Again, never treat a patient with foreign body sensation with topical anesthetic in order to permit him or her to continue the sports activity.

Subconjunctival Hemorrhage

Blood beneath the conjunctiva looks quite red. It is often related to the breakage of a small blood vessel between the conjunctiva and the sclera. Although the injury may be related to severe trauma, it often is not. Usually the athlete has no complaints, other than the appearance of the eye. In the presence of a normal screening examination, a subconjunctival hemorrhage does not require therapy. If there is decreased visual acuity, a loss of the visual field in one area, irregularity of the pupils or pain, the athlete should be referred for more definitive evaluation and therapy. If the injury is related to blunt trauma, but none of the warning signs of internal injury exists, it is still wise to have the eye examined by an ophthalmologist within 24 hours. The subconjunctival hemorrhage itself generally disappears over a time course similar to that of a bruise of the skin, with similar color changes lasting approximately two weeks.

Serious Injuries Requiring Immediate Referral to Hospital Emergency Room or Ophthalmologist

Hyphema

A hyphema is defined as internal hemorrhage in the eye, which can be seen covering over a portion of the iris.[4] Therefore, this blood is between the cornea and the iris. A small amount of blood is not damaging, but trauma severe enough to create a hemorrhage can cause associated injuries in the eye. This type of injury is usually caused by blunt trauma and the athlete usually has a red aching eye. Visual acuity usually is decreased and can be measured on the near card. This injury is very serious, and is prone to rebleeding and internal damage to the eye; therefore, it should be seen and treated by a medical eye physician. The first-aid giver should **not** administer aspirin, as this can have the effect of increasing the rebleed rate.

Orbital Bone Fracture

Fractures of the bones of the orbit include pure blow-outs, which do not involve the orbital rim, as well as more complicated fractures that do. These patients usually look as if they have a black eye, with some limitation of eye movement, and some swelling of the lid. Often, there is a history of blunt trauma to the face. If the athlete does have limitation of eye movements, or if the globe is protruding from or sunken into the head, there may be some serious damage, requiring evaluation by a medical eye physician.

Ruptured (Open) Globe

This type of injury is one of the most serious in the realm of sports eye trauma. It can be caused by blunt trauma, in which the globe is ruptured, or by sharp injury, in which case the eye may be lacerated or penetrated. Usually, the size and shape of the pupil are irregular, and vision is decreased. The eye may also be red and there may be an associated hyphema. The diagnosis of an open globe is not as easy as it would seem. Often the injury can be subtle or missed, especially in a case of a laceration of the eyelid. Most people will not manipulate the lacerated lid and therefore will not adequately inspect the globe. It is best to protect this eye with a shield, without putting any pressure on the globe. No medications should be instilled into the eye. This injury is an extreme emergency, and the patient should be seen immediately by a medical eye physician (ophthalmologist).

Corneal Abrasion

Often this injury is signaled by sharp eye pain of sudden onset. It may be that the eye was poked with a finger (basketball), leading to severe tearing, photophobia, and a red eye. Patching the eye closed with the pad may provide great relief. In experienced hands, the diagnosis can be made by placing a wet fluorescein strip against the conjunctiva and allowing the color to wash across the cornea. The area of abrasion will stain (green) with the fluorescein dye and should be visible with a penlight. Topical anesthetic may be helpful in the diagnosis by relieving the pain, but should **never** be used as a treatment to allow the athlete to continue the sport.

Corneal Foreign Body

A corneal foreign body produces a history and symptoms similar to those of a corneal abrasion. Often, however, there is not the immediately preceding finger scratch to the eye. The athlete may say that something suddenly flew into his/her eye. Upon inspection with a penlight, often it is possible to see the foreign body lodged on the surface of the cornea. Experienced personnel may try a drop of topical anesthetic, followed by squeeze bottle irrigation, in an attempt to dislodge the foreign body. If the foreign body does become dislodged, then the patient should be treated as having a corneal abrasion.

Unfortunately, some foreign bodies penetrate the cornea and do not sit superficially. **Never** try to wipe off a *corneal* foreign body. The cornea is very thin (1/2 mm) and it is possible to push the foreign body through the cornea and into the eye. This injury is much more safely handled by a trained medical eye physician.

Lid Laceration

Lacerations of the eyelid are usually the result of a sharp injury. Consequently, there is usually bleeding from the eyelid and the eyelid function may be decreased. Repairing eyelid lacerations is best left to the skill of an ophthalmologist. Inappropriate closure of the laceration involving the margin of the eyelid can leave the patient with a disabling and disfiguring eyelid. Please be aware that eyelid lacerations may hide lacerations of the eyeball itself.

A Major Medical Emergency: Chemical Burn

The rapidity with which a chemical (acid or base) may burn through the exterior coats of the eye and damage the internal structures is quite alarming. The damage is caused so fast that emergency treatment with copious fluid irrigation of the damaged eye is necessary immediately at the time and place of the injury. Best vision results if irrigation begins within five minutes of injury.

Almost any fluid readily available can help to wash and save the eye. The first-aid provider should forcibly hold the eyelids open, so that the irrigating fluid flows directly over the globe. The irrigation should be continued for a minimum of five minutes by the clock. Ten is better. If the emergency room is a half hour away, irrigate a good twenty minutes by the clock before transporting the injured athlete. Get someone to help you. Make sure the athlete's hands and face are clean of any chemical. Ask your aide to call the emergency room, give the athlete's name, and say that the eye has been burned by the specific chemical, if known. Do not cover the eye with a pad or shield.

SUMMARY

An eye injury while participating in sports is a devastating way for a health conscious individual to have his or her lifestyle altered. Fortunately, the vast majority of sports-related ocular injuries can be prevented if the proper eye protection, in combination with a head protector (as needed), is used. Different sports have different risk factors for eye injuries, and athletes whose vision in their worst eye would not allow them to obtain a driver's license should be aware, not only of the risk factors, but of the eye protectors available. Athletes with eye conditions predisposing to injury should consider low-risk sports and use the appropriate eye protector whenever possible.

First-aid for eye injuries involves repeating the eye screening examination for comparison with the preinjury report. Patients who have deficits in visual acuity, visual field, pupillary exam, or motility examination should be referred for specialty care. Likewise, athletes with foreign bodies need care by medical eye physicians. Disorders treatable by first-aid personnel include lost or dislodged contact lenses, conjunctival foreign bodies, "black eye," and conjunctival hemorrhage. Chemical burns to the eye should be treated immediately at the location of injury, prior to referral for definitive care.

Table 13-3

DISPOSITIONS ACCORDING TO SYMPTOMS AND SIGNS

Symptoms and Signs	Possible Diagnosis	Disposition
Chemical in eye	Chemical corneal burn	Flush with any fluid for 10 minutes by the clock, then immediately to emergency room

(continued)

Symptoms and Signs	Possible Diagnosis	Disposition
Blurred vision (not cleared with blinking)	Corneal abrasion; hyphema; internal eye injury	Pad and refer to ophthalmologist
Blurred vision (normal with blinking)	Mucus in the eye	Irrigate
Deficiency in visual field	Retinal detachment	Refer to ophthalmologist
Pain (sharp, stabbing)	Corneal foreign body	Pad and refer to ophthalmologist
Pain (deep, throbbing)	Iritis; acute glaucoma	Refer to ophthalmologist
Double vision	Nerve damage; muscle trauma; blowout fracture	Refer to ophthalmologist
Light sensitivity (white eye)	Contusion	Ice to the eye
Rainbows around lights after swimming	Corneal edema (chemical toxicity)	Do nothing, wait
Foreign body sensation or scratchiness in the eye	Dislodged contact lens; conjunctival foreign body	See text under "Emergency Eye Kit"
Itching	Allergy	Irrigate
Tearing (comfortable eye)	Infection	Antibiotic and hand washing
Black eye with pain or bleeding or blurred vision	Blowout fracture; internal injury	Refer to ophthalmologist
Black eye (isolated)	Contusion	Ice for 24 hours
Foreign body on the cornea	Corneal foreign body	Refer to ophthalmologist
Foreign body on sclera	Conjunctival foreign body	See text
Decreased motility	Paresis; blowout fracture; muscle damage	Refer to ophthalmologist
Proptosis (bulging eye)	Orbital hemorrhage	Refer to ophthalmologist
Abnormal pupil	An open globe hyphema or internal injury	Shield and refer to ophthalmologist (No pad)
Blood on the iris or pupil	Hyphema	Refer to ophthalmologist (Do not give aspirin)
Cut eyelid	Lid laceration	Shield and refer to ophthalmologist
Cut sclera	Open globe	Shield and refer to ophthalmologist (No pad)
Disorganized eye	Ruptured globe	Shield and refer to ophthalmologist (No pad)

REFERENCES

1. Vinger, P.F.: The eye and sports medicine. Chapter 45. In Duane, T.D. (ed.): *Clinical Ophthalmology.* Philadelphia, Harper and Row, revised 1984, Vol. V, pp. 1-51.
2. *The Athlete's Eye: Ophthalmology in Sports.* San Francisco, CA, American Academy of Ophthalmology, 1982.
3. Gombos, G.M.: *Handbook of Ophthalmic Emergencies.* Flushing, N.Y., Medical Examination Publishing Company, 1973.
4. Pavan-Langston, D. (ed.): *Manual of Ocular Diagnosis and Therapy.* Boston, Little, Brown, 1985.

AUTHOR INDEX

A

Abramson, David H., v, xiii, 71
Adler, F H., 7
Aho, J., 148
Akssamit, G., 137
Albaugh, C.H., 66, 70
Albert, D.M., 121
Ali, Mohammed, 68
Allen, Merril J., 21, 43
Amyot, Marcel, v, xiii, 149, 170
Anderson, R.R., 43
Antaki, S., 170
Appleton, B., 27
Arbanas, Fred, 62
Ashe, Arthur, 100, 105, 106

B

Bahill, A. Terry, 6, 7, 126, 131
Bard, C., 109
Barsness, John, 148
Basu, P.K., 80
Benson, W.E., 66, 70
Berens, C., 121
Bing, Dave, 5
Binsborg, B., 109
Blais, Capt. B.R., 27
Block, Seymor S., 80
Bonifide, 128
Borg, Bjorn, 86, 100, 101
Bowen, D.I., 146, 148
Brancazio, Peter, 131
Bickford, W., 27
Brister, Bob, 148
Brody, Howard, 92, 94, 95
Burns, Stanley, 66, 67, 70

C

Caldwell, G.G., 80
Calvin, M., 121
Campbell, F.W., 7
Castren, J., 148
Chapman, Seville, 125
Chevaleraud, J.P., 170
Chisholm, L.D.J., 170
Clark, John William, 80
Clarke, N.A., 80
Cole, M., 68, 70
Conigliaro, 131
Connors, Jimmy, 86, 103
Cotter, J., 79, 80
Crawford, J.S., 170
Cullen, A.P., 32, 33, 43
Cullen, J., 80

D

Daroff, R.B., 109
Davis, John K., v, xiii, 9, 27
Dimaio, V.J.M., 148
Ditchburn, R., 109
Doggart, James, H., 66, 70
Drummond, J., 146, 148
Drye, J.C., 148
Duane, Thomas D., 43, 185
Duckworth, W.H., 11, 43
Duke, M., 109
Duke-Elder, S., 148, 170
Dumas, J., 170

E

Easterbrook, W.M., 109

Eaton, Scott, 5
Eifrig, D.E., 27
Ellis, George S., Jr., v, xiii, 171
Evert, Chris, 100

F

Fair, Gordon M., 80
Fender, D., 109
Fleury, M., 109
Fry, G.A., 27
Fujishiro, T., 109

G

Gattuso, Lorraine, xi
Gazenko, O.G., 121
Gerulaitus, Vitas, 86, 93
Getz, D.J., 137
Gieser, R.G., 80
Gombos, G.M., 185
Gregg, James R., 148
Guerry, D., III., 29, 43
Guerry, R.K., 29, 43

H

Haag, J.R., 80
Hackett, D., 121
Haik, Barrett G., iii, v
Helveston, Eugene M., v, xiii, 51
Ham, W.T., Jr., 29, 43
Hammer, Mark J., 80
Head, Howard, 92, 94
Heath, Donald, 121
Hedgecock, L.W., 80
Hoefle, Frank B., vi, xiii, 4, 7, 123
Hoffman, L.G., 109
Holter, N., 109
Hoshikawa, H., 109
Hubel, D.H., 4, 6, 7
Husak, W., 137

J

Jabar, Kareem Abdul, 5
Jacobson, R.I., 80
Jonasson, F., 80
Jones, Melville G., 7
Jones, Michael J., 7
Jordan, Barry D., vi, xiii, 65

K

Keeney, Arthur H., 27
Kieler, R.A., 148
Kim, Kyung, 68, 70
King, Billy Jean, 106
Kirsch, Anne, xi
Kojovic, V., 148
Kors, Kermit, 11, 43
Krysiewicz, Alice, xi

L

Labelle, Pierre F., vi, xiii, 149, 170
LaMarre, David A., 11, 43
Lapinski, Patricia, xi
LaRitz, Tom, 7, 131
Leigh, R. John, 7
Lensen, 73
Leonard, Sugar Ray, 66, 67
Levin, Daniel B., 70
Lieberman, Theodore, 66, 67, 70
Little, J.M., 170
Lubin, J.R., 121
Lundberg, G.D., 70

M

MacDaniel, Donald, 148
Macguire, J.I., 66, 70
Mackay, Cynthia, vi, xiii, 45
Magauran, D., 148
Mahoney, 73
Martone, W.J., 80
Mayne, S., 109
McDonough, Richard A., IV, vi, xiii, 71
McEnroe, John, 90, 103
Midorikawa, C., 109
Milder, Benjamin, 148
Mohler, S.R., 121
Moore, Sally, vi, xiii, 3
Morehouse, C.R., 13, 14
Moriority, Helen, xi
Moses, Robert A., 121
Moss, Hugh M., vi, xiii, 3
Mueller, H.A., 29, 43

N

Nastase, Ilie, 103
Navratilova, Martina, 106

O

Ogle, K.N., 7
Okun, Daniel A., 80

P

Page, Warren, 148
Palmer, Arnold, 133
Palmer, Edward, 66, 67, 70
Parrish, J.A., 29, 43
Pashby, R.C., 170
Pashby, Thomas J., 160, 170
Pavan-Langston, D., 185
Perchel, G., 170
Petstonic, A., 80
Pitts, D.G., 28, 29, 32, 33, 43
Pizzarello, Louis D., iii, vi, xiii, 7, 65
Plante, Jacques, 163
Purisic, S., 148

R

Ramanan, S., 109
Reeve, T.G., 137
Renne, D., 121
Richards, J. Rodney, 127
Roberts, A.H., 70
Roberts, Calvin W., vii, xiii, 133
Robertson, D.M., 147, 148
Rosenfield, A.R., 11, 43
Ross, Ronald J., 68, 70
Rouse, M., 109
Rousseau, Alain P., vii, xiii, 149, 170, 171
Rubin, Melvin L., 148
Ruffolo, J.J., Jr., 29, 43
Rutanen, H., 148
Ryan, J.B., 109

S

Softly, Bill, 67
Salisbury, James A., vii, xiii, 139
Sankett, 73
Schalen, L., 7
Schuster, G., 148
Score, 131
Sheppard, B., 121
Slatt, Bernard J., vii, xiii, 81
Sliney, David H., 26, 27, 29, 43

Smith, Hunter, 61
Stein, Harold A., vii, xiii, 81
Stein, Raymond M., vii, xiii, 81
Stelland, 68
St. Helen, Roger, 11, 43
St. Yves, 159

T

Takahashi, M., 109
Tanner, Roscoe, 100
Tauber, Gil, 131
Telcher, Elliot, 85
Thompson, J., 68, 70
Tolpin, D.W., 109

U

Urbach, R., 43

V

Verdenthal, 69
Viessman, Warren, Jr., 80
Vinger, Paul F., 13, 36, 43, 109, 130, 131, 160, 161, 170, 185
Von Allen, Maurice, 70

W

Walker, Wesley, 4
Wannebo, M., 137
Watson, Tom, 133, 134
Weidenthal, Daniel T., 70
Whiteside, T.C.D., 121
Whiteson, A.L., 70
Whitmore, Wayne M., vii, xiii, 111
Wiedman, M., 152, 170
Wiesel, T.N., 4, 7
Wigglesworth, E.C., 11, 12, 43
Williams, David R., 121
Wolbarsht, Myron, 43
Wolfe, S.M., 66, 70
Woolley, Robert, xi
Wright, W.L., 80
Wurtz, R.H., 7

Z

Zee, David S., 7
Zimmerman, L.E., 66, 70

SUBJECT INDEX

A

Actinic conjunctivitis, among baseball players, 130
Actinic keratoconjunctivitis
  conditions due to, 27
  induction of, 27
Alcohol, color blindness associated with, 48
Allyl resin
  fracture energy studies, 14, 15
  mean fracture energies, table, 12
  properties of, table, 34
  use of lens material, 10
  weight, thickness and index factors, table, 33
Amateur Hockey Association of the U.S., standards for eye protection, 13
Amblyopia
  concern for second eye, 4-5
  eye protection needed by football player with, 59
  eye-hand coordination and, 4
American Society for Testing Materials
  eye protection in sports studies, 13-14
    for hockey, 13
    for youth baseball, 14
    results, table, 14
    standards set, 13, 41
Ammetropia
  correction of in baseball players
    contact lenses, 129-130
    spectacles, 128-129
  spectacles issued to Mets players, 128-129
Aquatic sports, 71-79
  adjustments to water made, 71
  banned eye drops, 79
  chlorine (*see* Chlorine)
  effects on the eye, 75-79

eye infections related to chlorine, 76-79 (*see also* Chlorine)
ocular irritation from swimming pools, 75-79
  chlorine irritation, 75
  corneal abrasions, 75
  corneal edema, 75
  mechanical factors, 76
  types of, 75
scuba diving, 79
swimming pool disinfection, 72-75
  chlorine (*see* Chlorine)
  organisms killed, table, 73
  pH factor and, 72, 74
  purpose of, 74
  use bromine, 75
  use iodine, 74-76
  use of goggles, 79
Artificial sweeteners, ultraviolet sensitivity and, 30
Auto racing
  eye and face protection recommended, table, 173
  risk factors, table, 173
Aviation ophthalmology, 111-120
  aerobatics, 111
  aviation as transportation, 111
  aviation for sport, 111
  effect high altitude flying on visual function, 117
    use of oxygen, 117
  effects of glare, 114
  eye changes at high altitudes, 118
  eye injuries causes, 118
  movement as three dimensional in aircraft, 112
  night vision, 114-115
    use red lighting in cockpit, 116
  pilot visual illusions, 115-116

autokinesis, 115
oculogravic, 115-116
poor pilot performance factors, 118
regulations, 112-114 (*see also* Federal Aviation Regulations)
resistance to effects acceleration, 116-118
  area of least tolerance, 117
  factors in, 116
  lines of least resistance, 117
  results, graph, 116
  use G-suit, 117
  use of oxygen, 117-118
situational lighting and optical illusions, 114-116
use peripheral vision, 114

B

BB shooting, eye protection recommended, 39
Baseball ophthalmology, 123-131
  actinic conjunctivitis and, 130
  catcher's visual demand, 124
  conclusions, 131
  correction of ammetropia (*see also* Ammetropia)
    contact lenses, 128-129 (*see also* Contact lenses)
    spectacles, 128
  eye injuries and medical problems
    common problems, 130-131
    incidence, 130, 171
  eye protection recommended, 14, 33
  face protection recommended, table, 173
  risk factors, table, 173
  fielding visual demands, 123-124
    velocity of pitched ball, 123
  infielder visual demand, 124-125
    use contact lens, 124-125
  outfielder visual demand, 125
    trigonometric theory of fielding balls, 125
  pitcher visual demands, 124
    use glasses and contact lenses, 124
  tension symptoms 131
  visual acuity demand in hitting, 126
    following ball visually, 126
    use of glasses, 126
  visual demands in baseball, 123
    catchers, 124
    fielding, 123
    hitting, 126
    infielders, 124-125
    outfielders, 125
    pitchers, 124
  youth
    eye and face protection recommended, 14, 33, 39
    faceguard standards, 41
Basketball
  eye protection recommended, 39
  risk factors, table, 173
Bird shooting, eye protection recommended, 39
Boxing (*see* Pugilism)
Brain injury, in boxing, 68
Bromide, swimming pool disinfection using, 75
Bromochlordimethydantoin, swimming pool disinfection using, 75
Broomball, injuries due to, 160

C

CR 39 (*see* Allyl resin)
Cataract
  color blindness due to, 47-48
  tennis related, 97
  traumatic, boxing related, 66
Chemical burn of eye, immediate care, 182-183
Chloramphenical, color blindness due to, 47
Chlorine
  biocidial effects of on organisms, 75, 78
    table, 77
  combined available chlorine defined, 72
  disinfection of swimming pools using, 72-75
    enzyme trace substance theory, 74
    organisms killed, table, 73, 77
    purpose, 74
    role pH factor, 72, 74
    safe area for chlorination, 78
  eye infections related to chlorine, 76-79
    conjunctivitis (*see* Conjunctivitis)
    control of Adenovirus, 78, 79
  due chlorine, 76-79 (*see also* Chlorine)
  eye irritation in swimmers due to, 75-76
    and chloramines, 75-76
  reaction in water, 71-72
  toxic effects of, 76-79
    table, 77

Choroidal rupture
  cause, 157
  illustration, 158
  results, 157
Climatic Droplet Keratopathy, 27
Collyrium with Ephedrine eye drops, 79
Color blindness, 46
  acquired, 47
  blue yellow, 46
  causes of, 47-48
  cone monochromats, 46
  effect cataracts on, 47-48
  lenses recommended, 49
  red-green, 46-47
    cause, 46
    effect on occupations, 47
    incidence, 46
    tests for, 47
    transmission of, 46-47
  summary, 49
Cone monochromatic, definition, 46
Conjunctivitis
  and baseball players, 130
  of swimmers, 76, 78
    airborne and direct transmission, 79
    cause, 76
    epidemics reported, 78
    factors in, 76
    manifestations, 78
    prevention, 79
Color vision, 45-49
  causes of, 45
  color blindness (see Color blindness)
  cones needed for normal, 46
  factors in selection color ball used in racquet ball, 48
  in animals, 46
  in baseball players, 128
  lens best for glare intolerance, 49
  make-up of daytime eye, 45-46
  make-up of night time eye, 45-46
  purpose of, 45
  selection color for sunglasses, 48-49
Contact lenses
  hard versus soft lenses, 54-55
  treating lost and dislodged lens, 179
    disposition, table, 184
    symptoms, table, 184
  use of
    by baseball players, 124, 124-125, 129-130

  by football players, 54-55
  by hockey players, 153
  for shooting, 142
Corneal edema
  from swimmers, 75
  symptoms and disposition, table, 184
Cross-country skiing
  eye protection recommended, table, 173
  risk factors, table, 173
Cycling
  eye protection recommended, 39
  risk factor, table, 173
  table, 173

D

Digotin, color blindness due to, 47
Diplopia
  adaptation young children to, 5
  effect on athlete, 5
Diving (see Aquatic sports)
  eye trauma due to, 79
  goggles recommended, 39
  masks recommended, 39
Dress prescription glasses, lens materials used, 10

E

Eight Ball Syndrome, 154
Emergency eye kit, 177
  advanced, 177
    components of, table, 177
  basic, 177-178
    components, table, 177
Encephalopathy
  cause of, 68
  chronic traumatic type, 68
  syndrome symptoms, 68
Ethambutol, color blindness due to, 47
Eye protection for sports players
  lenses for (see Lens)
  recommended applications, 39-40
  standards for, 41
Eye injuries
  annual incidence, 171
    preventative injuries, 171
  associated with pugilism (see Pugilism)
  associated with shooting, 146-147
  baseball related, 130-131 (see also Baseball)

dispositions by symptoms and signs, table, 183-184
emergency eye kit (*see* Emergency eye kit)
first aid (*see* First aid)
hockey related, 153-158
lacerated eyelid, 59
ocular injuries
  disposition of, 179-183
  from swimming pools, 75
prevention (*see* Prevention of sports eye injuries)
related to flying, 118
serious injuries requiring immediate expert care, 180-183
  chemical burn, 182-183
  corneal abrasion, 181-182
  corneal foreign body, 182
  hyphema, 180-181
  lid laceration, 182
  orbital bond fracture, 181
  ruptured globe, 181
skiing related, 159-160
subconjunctival hemorrhage, 180
summary, 183
tennis related, 97
treatable by first aid personnel
  conjunctival foreign body, 179-180
  lost/dislodged contact lens, 179
  subconjunctival hemorrhage, 180
Eye-hand coordination in sports
  amblyopia and, 4-5
  detection of motion and, 3-4
  sensory arc of, 3-4

F

Face protector for hockey
  as requirement to play, 160-161
  design of, 164
    approvals of, 164-165
    illustration, 165
  effectiveness of, 161
  molded, for goaltenders, 163
    illustration, 163
  polycarbonate type, 166
    illustration, 166
    visual field, illustration, 167
  publicity regarding, 161
    illustration, 162
  purpose, 164
  vision while wearing, 166
    computerized visual field, illustration, 167
  visor for referees, 163
    illustration, 164
  wire-mesh type, 164, 165
    illustration, 165
  visual fields, illustration, 167
Federal Aviation Regulations, 112-114
  First-class medical certificate
    use of, 113
    visual requirements, 112, 113, 119
  Second-class medical certificate
    use of, 113
    visual requirements, 112, 119-120
  Third-class medical certificate, 112, 120
    use of, 113
  use of oxygen, 117
  visual requirements, 112, 119-120
    color vision needed, 113
    for First-class medical certificate, 119
    for Second-class medical certificate, 119-120
    for Third-class medical certificate, 120
    near vision requirements, 113
    use of glasses, 113
    visual fields required, 114
Fencing
  face protection recommended, table, 173
  risk factor, table, 173
First aid for sports injuries (*see also* Eye injuries)
  emergency eye kit, 177-178
  football trainers sideline kit contents, 62
  injuries treatable by, 179-180
  serious injuries requiring professional care, 180-183
  useful techniques, 178
Fishing
  eye protection recommended, table, 173
  risk factor, table, 173
  selection color for sunglasses, 49
Floor hockey
  injuries due to, 160
  protectors to prevent, 39
Football, 51-64
  amblyopia, 59
  eye care first aid kit contents, 62
  eye examination for players, 52-54, 64
    baseline criteria for, 52
    extensiveness of, 53-54

form used, example, 53
  ocular histories needed, 54
eye injuries related to, 59
eye protection recommended, 39
head protection recommended, table, 173
  risk factor, table, 173
importance care of "black eye," 62, 64
monocular vision, 62
nonglare cream use on cheeks, 63
  illustration, 63
ocular motility of players, 57-58, 64
  depth perception, 57-58
  stereopsis, 57-58
retinal disease, 58-59, 64
summary, 64
use of cage type face guard, illustration, 60
use of contact lenses by players, 54-55, 64
  hard versus soft, 54-55
use of face mask, 59, 61-62
  illustration, 60
  problem with, 62
  with plastic shield, illustration, 61
use of spectacles, 55
  Liberty Goggles®, 56
  Rec Specs®, 56
visual acuity needed, 57, 64
visual needs and position played, 51-52, 64
visual requirements for playing, 51-52
Foreign body in eye
  disposition, table, 184
  symptoms, table, 184
  treated by first aid personnel, 179-180
    techniques used, 180

G

G-Suit, use of, 117
Game hunting, eye protection recommended, 39
Glass blowers cataract, cause of, 31, 32
Glass lens, heat-treated
  mean fracture energies of, 12-13
    studies of, 14, 15
    table, 12
  properties of, table, 34
  use as lens material, 10, 11
  weight, thickness and index factors, table, 33
Glaucoma
  color blindness due to, 48

related to boxing injury, 66
tennis related, 97
Golf ophthalmology, 133-137
  advantages colored golf balls, 136
  determination ball location, 133
    changes due to glasses, 134
    examples, 134
  eye protection recommended, table, 173
    risk factor, table, 173
  planning golf swing, 134-135
  putting and visual acuity, 135-136
  role of vision in golf, 133
  visual acuity and head movement, 134-135
  visually handicapped golfers, 136-137

H

Handball
  ball velocity and impact energy study, 13
    table, 14
Head ski, developer of, 92
Hockey
  eye and face protection recommended, 39
    standards, 41
  eye injuries due to playing, 153-158, 171
    causes, 153
    hyphema, 154
    incidence and results, table, 157, 171
    late complications, 157
    perforating injuries, 156
    posterior segment injuries, 156-157
  face protectors used (see also Face protectors)
  floor hockey injuries, 160
  goalers face protection, 163
    molded face mask, illustration, 163
  head protection recommended, table, 174
    risk factor, table, 174
  hyphemic injuries, 154
    eight-ball syndrome, 154
    follow-up examination, 154
    illustration, 155
  ocular injury prototypic victim, 153
  optical tolerances of standards
    for plano protectors, table, 18
    for prescription lenses, table, 18
  perforating injuries, 156
    emergency treatment, 156
    illustration, 156
  posterior segment injuries, 156-157
    choroidal rupture, 157

illustration, 158
retinal detachment, 157
subretinal hemorrhages, 157
treatment, 157
types of, 156
prevention of eye injuries, 160-161, 169-170, 171-172
  effectiveness of program, 161
  extent of problem, 160
  publicity regarding, illustration, 162
  rule changes made, 160
  to goalers, 163
  to referees, 163
  to spectators, 164
  wearing face protector, 160, 161, 164-168
protection of spectators, 164
  use glass protectors around rink, 164
referees face protection, 163
visor, illustration, 164
soft tissue injuries, 154
visual requirements, 149, 152-153
  adjustment for blind players, 150
  use contact lenses, 153
Horseback riding
head and eye protection recommended, 39
  risk factor, table 174
  table, 174
Hyphema
boxing related, 66
cause of injury, 180
consequences possible, 62
definition, 180
disposition, table, 183
hockey related, 154
  illustration, 155
symptoms, table, 183
tennis related, 97

I

INH, color blindness due to, 47
Ice hockey, eye protection standard, 13, 39, 41
Industrial safety glasses
lens materials used, 10
optical tolerances of standards
  for plano protectors, table, 18
  for prescription lenses, table, 18
requirements for, 11
Industrial Safety Standards

requirements for lens materials, 11
of mean fracture energy, table, 12
Infrared radiation, 31-32
divisions of spectrum, 31
effect temperature on spectrum of emission, 31
heating effect of concerns, 31
industrial standards for retinal protection, 31
range for concern for sports environment, 31
sources exposures to, 32-33
swimming pool disinfection using, 74-75
tennis related, 97

J

Jogging (see Running)

K

Keratoconjunctivitis, ultraviolet and, 30

L

Labrador Droplet Keratopathy, 27
Lacrosse, head protection recommended, table, 174
Lanoxin (see Digoxin)
Lenses for sports vision, 9-42
equiping oneself and decision making, 37-38
Food and Drug Administration rules for, 147
fracture energy studies, 13-14
Industrial Safety Standard for, 11
infrared radiation (see Infrared radiation)
lens materials and their impact resistance, 10-16
  allyl resin (see Allyl resin)
  dress prescription lenses, 10
  for industrial safety plano lenses, 10-11
  glass, heat treated (see Glasses)
  polycarbonate (see Polycarbonate)
levels of performance and protection eyewear, 35-36
litigation due broken spectacles, case examples, 15, 16
matching products to needs, 33-36
  lens materials compared, 33-35

levels performance and protection of sports eyewear, 35-36
problems with polycarbonate, 35
materials used compared, 33
weight, thickness, index factors, table, 33
measurement failure levels, 11-13
and speed of blows, 12-13
table, 12
measurement impact energy, 11-13
table, 12
optics and visual performance in sports (see Optics and visual performance)
polaroid used for shooting, 142
properties and product types lens materials, table, 34
protection from eye injury, 9-10
requirements for, 9
sports sunglasses (see Sunglasses)
sunglasses (see Sunglasses)
thickness of, 10, 11
tinted used for shooting, 141
ultraviolet radiation (see Ultraviolet radiation)
weight, thickness, index factors of, table, 33
Lenticular opacities, 27
Liberty Goggles
use by football players, 55
illustration, 56

M

Macular degeneration, color blindness due to, 48
Motorcycling, eye protection recommended, 39
Mountaineering, eye protection recommended, 39
Multiple sclerosis, color deficiency associated with, 48

N

Naphcon-A eyedrops, 79

O

Optics and visual performance in sports, 16-22
plano power protectors (see Plano power protectors)
prescription lens, 18-22 (see also Prescription lens)
Oral contraceptives, ultraviolet sensitivity and, 30

P

Pinqueculum, 27
Plano power protectors
goal of designers, 17
negative power advantages 16-17
optical tolerances of standards for, 18
table, 18
thickness lenses used, 33
with face form angle, illustration, 17
wrap around effect, 17, 18
Polarizing glass prescription lenses, 25
use of, 49
Polaroid, stereograms, 5
Polo, head and eye protection recommended, table, 174
Polycarbonate
advantages of use, 34-35
brain injury affecting visual system, 68
indirect effects, 68
symptoms increased intracranial pressure, 68
types of, 68
fracture energy studies, 14, 15
impact resistance of, 10
mean fracture energies, 12-13
table, 12
problems with, 35
properties of, table, 34
recommended use, 40
use as lens material, 10
weight, thickness and index factors, table, 33
Prefin, 79
Prefin-A eye drops, 79
Prescription lens
absorptive lens, 21-22
luminance transmittance, 22
design quality, 19
factory quality, 19
fitting quality, 20-21
fitting geometry of frame, illustration, 20
laboratory contribution to quality, 19-20
luminance transmittance, 22
materials used for, 10

optical tolerances of standards for, 18
performance of, 19
summary error sources and their effects, 21
sunglasses
  problems with prescription lens, 23-24
  tinted lens, 24-26
Prevention sports eye injuries
  effectiveness protective eye gear, 173
  first aid (see First aid for sports injuries)
  in monocular persons, 172-173
  post injury screening, 176-177
  preparticipation screening, 174-176
  previous ocular injury or surgery, 172-173
  protective eye gear wear (see Protective eye wear)
  risk factors for various sports, table, 173
  tennis safety precautions, 98
Protective eye gear
  effectiveness of, 173
  for auto racers, table, 173
  for baseball players, 14, 33, 39
    faceguard standards, 41
    table, 173
  for fencing, 173
  for fishing, 173
  for floor hockey players, 39
  for football players, 39, 55, 59
  for golf, 173
  for horseback riding, 39
  for polo playing, 174
  hockey-related, 160-167
  monocular sighted, 5
  standards for, 41
  various sports, 13-14, 39-40
    table, 173
Prince racket
  development of, 92
  high velocity-return of, 94
Punch-drunk syndrome (see Encephalopathy, chronic traumatic)
Pugilism
  adnexal injuries, 67-68
    epiphora, 68
    orbital fractures, 67
    ringside treatment, 67
  face protection recommended, 173
    table, 173
  glaucoma related to injury, 66
  indications for terminating bout, 69

ocular injury due to, 65-67
  types of, 65, 66
prevention of eye injuries, 68-69
  decisions by ringside physician, 69
  periodic ophthalmological examinations, 68-69
  protective headgear, 69
  use thumbless glove for boxing, 69
retinal detachment following injury, 66 (see also Retinal detachment)
susceptibility to foreign objects in eye, 65
traumatic cataracts due to injury, 66
Psoralens, ultraviolet sensitivity and, 30
Pterygium, 27

R

Racket sport
  ball velocity and impact energy studies, 13
    results, table, 14
  benefits polycarbonate lens, 13
  eye injuries annually due to, 171
  eye protection, 13, 39
    standards, 41
    table, 174
  optical tolerance of standards
    for plano protectors, table, 18
    for prescription lenses, table, 18
Radial keratotomy
  need ophthalmologist consult prior active sports, 172
  risks of to athlete, 4
Random dot stereogram, 5
Rec Specs
  description, 55
  illustration, 56
  use by football players, 55
Refractive error, of football players (see Football)
Retina detachment
  boxing-related, 66
  disqualifying participation in sports, 58
  hockey related, 157
  ophthalmologist consultation prior active sports, 172
  symptoms and signs, table, 184
  treatment, 66-67, 157
Running
  eye protection recommended, table, 174
  risk factor, table, 174

Subject Index

S

Saccadic eye movements, 66
Safety glasses
  use by tennis players, 97
    features needed, 98
  use when discharging firearms, 147
Sailing, eye protection recommended, 39
Scuba diving (*see also* Aquatic sports)
  contact lens problems, 79
Skeet shooting, speed of target, 145
Shooting and the eye, 139-147
  aids in aiming, 141-144
  aiming, 139-146
    aids used, 141-144
    eye dominance, 140-141
    refraction, 139-140
    with various weapons, 144-146
  basic principles of aiming, 139-140
  eye dominance, 140-141
  eye injuries due BB, pellet, lead shot, 146-147
    damage caused, 146
    ocular perforation, 147
    prevention of, 147
    prognosis for vision, 146
  importance stock design, 143
  injury prevention, 147
    knowledge rules gun safety and etiquette, 147
    use safety glasses, 147
  injury treatment, 146
  open and aperture sights for aiming, 142-143
  pistol marksmanship, 145-146
    factors in, 146
    lens for presbyope, 145-146
    tapes unsuppressed eye, 146
  refraction and aiming, 139-140
  rifle sighting, 145
  scopes used for aiming, 143-144
    focusing of, 144
    mirage effect, 144
    mounting of, 144
  shotgun aiming, 144-145
  uniocular target sighting, 140
Shortstops Eyes (*see* Actinic conjunctivitis)
Skeet shooting, eye protection recommended, 39
Ski goggles, 168-169
  illustration, 168, 169
  vision while wearing, 168
  worn over glasses, 168
    illustration, 169
Ski racing, eye and head protection recommended, table, 174
Skiing
  Alpine
    eye protection recommended, 39
    standards, 41
  blind skiers, 149
  by monocular skiers, 152
  corneal abrasions, 159
  factors affecting, 152
  injuries due to playing, 159-160
    corneal abrasion, 159
    perforating injuries, 159
    posterior segment injuries, 160
    snow blindness, 159
  perforating injuries, 159
  posterior segment injuries, 160
  prevention of injuries, 160-161
  ski goggles (*see* Ski goggles)
  snow blindness, 159
  visual requirements, 149, 151-152
    color vision, 151
    illumination, 151
    stereopsis, 151
    visual field, 151
  weather and accidents, 152
Smoking, color blindness related to, 48
Snorkeling (*see* Aquatic sports)
Snow blindness
  causes, 159
  prevention of, 168
  treatment, 159
Snow mobiling
  head and eye protection recommended, 39
  risk factors, table, 174
Soccer
  eye protector recommended, 39, 174
  risk factor, table, 174
Softball
  eye protection recommended, 39, 174
  risk factor, table, 174
Spectacles
  for correction ammetropia, 128-129
  shooting, 141, 142
  sports sunglasses (*see* Sunglasses)
Spheroidal degeneration, 27

Sports eye injuries (*see* Eye injuries)
Sports sunglasses (*see* Sunglasses)
Sports vision, use of term, 37
Squash
  ball velocity and impact energy study, 13
    table, 14
  color ball used, 48
  eye protection recommended, table, 174
Street hockey, eye and face protection recommended, 39
Stereograms
  Polaroid, 5
  random dot, 5
Stereopsis
  athletic performance and, 5, 7
  clinical tests for, 5
Strabismus, eye-hand coordination and, 4
Subretinal hemorrhage, 156-157
  illustration, 158
  treatment, 157
Sulfonamides, ultraviolet sensitivity and, 30
Sunglasses
  classification categories, 22
  colors of tinted lenses, 25-26
    selection of, 24-25, 48-49
  definition, 22, 36-37
  intelligent use of, 22-26
  lens materials, 10
  Liberty Goggles, 56
  luminance levels of, 22-23
    typical scenes, table, 22
  matching activity to, 37-38
  optical tolerances of standards, 18
    for plano protector, table, 18
    for prescription lenses, table, 18
  polarizing glass prescription lenses, 25
  prescription lens problems, 23-24
    negative lens, illustration, 24
  Rec Specs, 55
    illustration, 56
  sports needing, 59
  standard requirements, 36-37
  thickness of, 10
Swimming (*see also* Aquatic sports)
  eye protection recommended, 39
    risk factor, table, 174

T

Tennis visual approach to winning, 81-109

  asphalt court, 100
  ball velocity and impact energy studied, 13
    table, 14
  cement courts, 99-100
  clay courts, 99
  colors and vision in, 102
  court surfaces, 98-101
    adjustment racket strings to, 101
    cement, 99-100
    clay, 99
    grass, 100-101
    pointers on, 101
  eye protection recommended, table, 174
    risk factor, table, 174
  impact ball on racket, 91-95, 107
    as nonvisual event, 91-92
    measurement of duration of, 95
    physics of, 92-94
  indoor versus outdoor tennis, 102
  injuries related to players, 95-97
    factors in, 96-97
    prevention, 96
    rate of, 96, 97
    singles and doubles players, 95-96
    types of, 97
  line disputes, 103-105, 108
    conventions to help determine, 104-105
    settling of, 105
    use electronic field, 105
  ocular saccades defined, 83
  outdoor tennis, 102
  physics of racket size, 92-95
    impact ball on racket, 92, 94
    oversize racket, 92
    velocity of ball, 94, 98
  requirements of singles player, 95
    eye protection, 96
  running, 89-91, 107
  safety precautions, 98
  sensory fatigue symptoms, 108
  slow versus fast game, 88-89, 107
  spatial orientation problems, 102-103
  summary, 107-109
  sun as a factor in, 102, 103
  tracking fast ball with eye, 83, 107
    speed of ball, 84, 86
    variables in, 83-84
    zone of fog, 86-87
  use oversize racket, 92, 107
  vision and moving target, 82-83, 108

closing eyes, illustration, 85
visual memory, 87-88, 107
wearing of glasses while playing, 105-107
  illustration, 106
wind factor in, 102, 103
zone of fog, 83, 86-87
  definition, 86
  reduction of, 87
Tennis elbow, cause of, 94
Tetracyclines, ultraviolet sensitivity and, 30
Thiazides, ultraviolet sensitivity and, 30

U

Ultraviolet radiation
  cumulative effects of, 32-33
    glass blowers cataract, 32
    infrared exposures, 32-33
  damage due to, 32
  effects drugs on sensitivity to, 30-31
  effects of, 27-28
  in the environment, 29-31
    indoor exposures, 30-31
    risks in varied activities, 30
    sources of ultraviolet, 29
  ocular effects of, 27-28
  recommendation, 28-29
  retina damage due to, 28-29
  sources of, 29
  spectrum, zones and areas of concern, 26
    divisions of, 26-27
  standard for sun glasses, 28-29

V

Vasocon-A eye drops, 79
Visual physiology
  amblyopia, 4
  central visual acuity and movement, 4
  diplopia and, 5
  eye-hand coordination, 3-4
  monocular adaption, 5
  retinal disparity and, 5
  saccadic eye movements, 6
  sensitivity retinal receptors to contrasts, 3
  sensitivity retinal surface to movement, 4
  sensory fusion and, 4
  stereopsis, 5, 7
  strabismus, 4
  summary, 6-7
  use protective eye wear, 5
  vergence eye movements, 6
  vestibulo-ocular reflexes, 6
Volleyball, eye protection recommendation, 39

W

Winter sports, 149-170
  conclusions, 169-170
  emergency eye kit (*see* Emergency eye kit)
  evolution of eye injuries past decade, 160-161
  hockey (*see* Hockey)
  injuries secondary to sport, 153-160
    blindness due to, table, 157
    number of, table, 157
    to hockey, 153-157
    to skiing, 159-160
  ocular injuries disposition, 179-183 (*see also* Eye injuries)
  postinjury screening, 176-177
  preparticipation screening, 174-176
    eye examination, 174-176
    medical history, 174
    visual acuity and fields, 175-176
  prevention of hockey related injuries, 160-167, 169-170
    evolution of past decade, 160-161
    to goalers, 163
    to referees, 163
    to spectators, 164
    use face protector, 164-167
  prevention ski-related injuries, 168-169
  skiing (*see* Skiing)
  visual requirements, 149-151

Z

Zincfrin eye drops, 79

NO LONGER THE PROPERTY
OF THE
UNIVERSITY OF R.I. LIBRARY